SPECIAL EDUCATIONAL NEEDS AND DISABILITY (SEND) IN UK SCHOOLS

Carrie Grant

SPECIAL EDUCATIONAL NEEDS AND DISABILITY (SEND) IN UK SCHOOLS

A parent's perspective

The Education Studies Collection

Collection Editor
Janise Hurtig

LPP

First published in 2022 by Lived Places Publishing

The authors and editors have made every effort to ensure the accuracy of information contained in this publication, but assumes no responsibility for any errors, inaccuracies, inconsistencies and omissions. Likewise, every effort has been made to contact copyright holders. If any copyright material has been reproduced unwittingly and without permission the Publisher will gladly receive information enabling them to rectify any error or omission in subsequent editions.

British Library Cataloguing in Publication Data
A CIP record for this book is available from the British Library

ISBN: 9781915271006 (pbk)
ISBN: 9781915271020 (ePDF)
ISBN: 9781915271013 (ePUB)

The right of Carrie Grant to be identified as the Author of this work has been asserted by her in accordance with the Copyright, Design and Patents Act 1988.

Cover design by Fiachra McCarthy
Book design by Rachel Trolove of Twin Trail Design
Typeset by Newgen Publishing UK

Lived Places Publishing
Long Island
New York 11789

www.livedplacespublishing.com

This book is dedicated to David and our children. Your stories are my world.

A message from the author

A message to the learners, the curious and those who care about our young people.

I, and many parents like me, are desperate for you to be the best educator you can be. We are willing you to lead in fully understanding our children and giving them the best education they can possibly get. We champion you from the sidelines to become all you can be, working alongside us, so our young people can become all they can be. For the future is in their hands.

Carrie Grant

A note on language

In this book, I have chosen to use the most up-to-date preferred language in the United Kingdom, which is identity-first language – for example, I describe my children on the ASC spectrum as autistic instead of as people with autism. I also use Autism Spectrum Condition (ASC) to avoid the "Disorder" of ASD (Autism Spectrum Disorder).

Abstract

This book explores the experience of children who have special educational needs and/or disabilities (SEND) in UK schools, from the perspective of a parent. Through recollecting and reflecting on her own experiences and the experiences of her four children, the author sets the scene of the current educational context; reflects on the necessity of leadership as a skill; explores how collaboration does and could work in a school setting; considers the purpose of an individual strategy for each child; recounts the tools and strategies that have worked for her children; and questions what the future of education might look like.

Keywords

SEND, SEN, Special Educational Needs, Education, Parent Participation, School Experience, Inclusion, Disability, Teaching, Diversity

Contents

Introduction

When they think of school, most people imagine a classroom with 30 children, a teacher, and a teaching assistant. Work is led from the front with the children listening, following, and working to a greater or lesser extent and at differing speeds. What we may not think about is that nearly one-fifth of the children in that class have Special Educational Needs (SEN) – also sometimes called Special Educational Needs and Disabilities (SEND). This could be a physical disability, a neurological difference, or a mental health challenge.

We also know that there are many children with SEN who are not in school, having been off-rolled[1] or permanently excluded. Add to this the 100,000 children in the United Kingdom who did not return to school after the pandemic, and it makes for an alarming landscape. SEN children have become collateral damage in the race of schools to get to the top of the league tables – or, at the very least, to avoid being shamed by finding themselves in the lower half of the league table.

This "all children learning happily together" image is the one I had when I started on my journey as a mum. I have four children, two in their twenties, one teen, and one pre-teen. Three are birth children and one was adopted, and all have additional needs, often referred to as Special Educational Needs. Even these words are problematic for me. My children are considered to have "needs" because they are outside the range of what is defined as "normal". But who decides what normal should look like? Our culture, history, traditions, faiths? What about children who are considered "normal" – do they not have needs too? Why are needs seen as a bad thing to have? Would my children still be considered "needy" if we redefined "normal" and broadened the definition a little?

In 1966, early studies of autism showed a prevalence of 4.5 per 10,000 children (Lotter, 1966). If we jump to 2013, that figure was shown to be one in 50 (Blumberg et al., 2013). It could be argued that if this prevalence continues to increase, autistic people could be the new "normal" – they would then be the predominant neurotype.

Not being able to fit into a neurotypical world means those who are neurodivergent will always be expected to change and cope, and will often need adjustments made for them. When something is judged as working for the majority, it is very hard to get institutions or wider society to open up their thinking and consider another, more inclusive way of doing things. The irony is that in my experience, the institution of school – the one that should be the most open to learning and change – is actually the most rigid of thinkers.

***

SEND in the United Kingdom

The concept of SEND was first talked about in the late 1970s, replacing the term "handicap" that was used in the 1944 Education Act (Hodkinson, 2015). The first Code of Practice came some 50 years later (DfE, 1994), so it has been a slow process. But what of teacher training in SEND? Until recently, Initial Teacher Training

(ITT) in the United Kingdom did not have to include autism training at all, and the time given for learning about *all* SEND was limited to approximately two days. The 2016 Framework of Core Content for Initial Teacher Training made this training mandatory in 2016, and embedded practice began in 2018 (DfE, 2016, p. 17).

We still have no compulsory SEND training for the police force and in a 2017 report, more than one-third of general practitioners (GPs) (39.5%) reported that they had never received formal training on autism – either during or after their qualifications (Unigwe et al., 2017). Learning disability and autism training for health and care staff is only now in the consultation stage. Even autism training for staff working with children in young people's mental health inpatient units only started being delivered in 2021 (DHSC, 2019).

***

When I started my parenting journey, I was just as unenlightened. I knew next to nothing about autism, Attention Deficit (Hyperactivity) Disorder (AD(H)D), adoption, dyslexia, dyspraxia, dyscalculia, non-binary gender identities, transmasculine identities, demi-girl identities, queer identities, gay identities, or dysphoria. I knew nothing of self-harm, suicidal ideation, absconding, or child-on-parent violence. I knew nothing of Special Education Needs Coordinators (SENCos), Child and Adolescent Mental Health Services (CAMHS), Local Authorities, or Education and Health Care Plans (EHCPs). I knew nothing of mainstream provision, reasonable adjustments, special schools, pupil referral units, or home education. I also knew nothing of the exclusion, the isolation, or the judgement that can accompany

any or all of these things. This book explores the stories of how I learned all about this stuff – often the hard way. In working with many parents and professionals over the years, as well as being a professional coach myself, my aim is to share and suggest – never to tell you what to do. These kinds of learning best happen by sharing best practice rather than rule making. So often I find myself saying, "Give me someone who knows more than me." I am desperate for insights from professional experts or experts by experience. And this is what I am: an expert by experience. I sincerely hope you have a few lightbulb moments while reading this book and, more than anything, I hope you take the lightbulb moments and expand them into beautiful experiences in your own landscape.

One final thought before we begin. This book describes everything I didn't know before becoming a parent to SEND children, and everything that you might not know about education for those with additional needs. What I do know, though, is equally important and worth remembering as you read the stories that follow: my family is incredible and my children are outstanding. My home is full of people – the people we have chosen to gather: the misfits, the marginalized, the creatives, the quirky. These are our people. Our village is in our home, and it works. We have joy, laughter, pain, tears, and a whole heap of mess. Our home is full of love, and acceptance, and the celebration of small wins. It is a culture of noticing every breakthrough, learning and growing, listening, and constantly evolving – for all of us, but crucially for us as parents, shapeshifting into everything we need to be to parent our amazing children.

Learning objective: Language about diversity

To begin to understand the breadth and depth of the diversity in humanity and the language used to talk about it, and to begin to develop a mindset of openness and curiosity.

1
The landscape

We live in a postmodern society. By this, I mean we live in a society that no longer adheres to one belief or one big-picture story.
If we understand there to be one overarching story, it follows that
we are all a part of that story: we all know our place in that story, we
perceive our history through the same lens as one another, we all
live by a shared moral code, we toe the line, and we understand
where we fit – whether it is fair and equal or not. During the late
nineteenth century and the early part of the twentieth century,
philosophers and psychologists were challenging the truths and
motivations that created the story of their time. These challenges
struck at the core of society's foundations, changing the way we
think and ultimately leading to a rise in new concepts of equality
and inclusion.

One story versus many stories

In our postmodern lives, we face a relatively new challenge.
Should we all live with an "each to their own" attitude? Do we
all hold an individualistic outlook that says, "This is my story.
This is my truth"? Perhaps the world of home-schooling may
have some of this underlying belief – I will explore my family's
experience of home education a little later in this book but, on
the surface, the idea of every child learning in their own home

feels very individualistic. Should we all return to the one story instead? The institution? It has always worked before, after all, so maybe we should return to "common sense". Or does the story need to be rewritten to include other voices, telling other stories that until now have not been heard – for instance, the feminist voice, the Black voice, the disabled voice, the LGBTIQ+ voice, and the neuro-divergent voice?

Bearing all of this in mind as we turn to the dialogue around SEND, you will hear the voices of these worldviews. You may notice the dominance of the "let's return to one story" voice. By raising the voices of those who were previously excluded, we threaten the status quo and challenge the perceived natural order. We make those leaders who have the one-story worldview feel as if their dominant voice is being threatened, and is at risk of being lost.

The increase in the number of children being diagnosed with SEND has led to many voices being raised that challenge the status quo. As you speak up on behalf of a child with SEND, here are some sentences you may hear in response:

> "We never had all these children with autism and AD(H)D when we were kids. There were kids who didn't fit in but we all just got on with it."
>
> "Why do we keep labelling these children?"
>
> "If parents got on with parenting properly we wouldn't have all these children misbehaving."
>
> "ADHD is just an excuse for bad parenting."
>
> "Generational trauma is causing this upsurge."
>
> "Diet is causing this upsurge."
>
> "The environment is causing this upsurge."

"Vaccines are causing this upsurge."

"Kids are spoilt and have no resilience, so they develop mental health problems."

"Kids need greater discipline."

"Smack them into submission."

"Neurodiversity is a sickness."

"Why should we make adjustments for your child – who do you think you are? Who do they think they are?"

"We cannot change. If we do it for one, we have to do it for all."

"The way we were educated worked for us before, so why can't we continue to educate in the same way?"

"I'm here to teach, not be a therapist."

"The problem is people with all these 'woke' ideas."

There is a battle going on between those who, for whatever reason, are invested in the status quo and those who are begging the system to adapt so their children can be included equally.

Equity versus equality

Let us not confuse equal provision with equality. Equality does not mean "the same". Equality may mean that my child needs more provision than yours – this is a concept sometimes called "equity".

This is an important difference, because sometimes it might appear that equitable and inclusive provision is not "equal", which can be upsetting for some and can lead to push-back. The world right now is geared towards the neurotypical – those

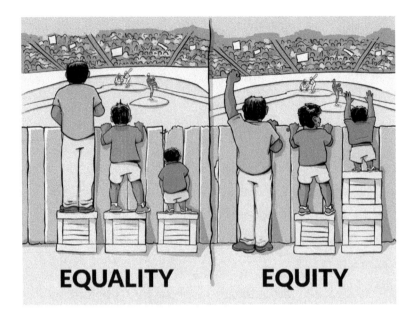

Figure 1 Equality vs. equity. Source: Interaction Institute for Social Change | Artist: Angus Maguire.

who have been declared "normal". When a group decides to reach for inclusion, the whole system changes – and this can feel uncomfortable for those who have always benefited from the system, because it can feel as if something is being taken away (whether or not it actually is). When those who feel challenged look at equitable provision, it can feel vastly unfair when they notice that it is not "equal" – that is, that they are not getting the same assistance as those who need more help. For the privileged, equity can feel like oppression.

Deconstruction is painful, and the institution of education may resist the challenge to its institutional thinking. But it is important: we cannot build something that works for everyone without first deconstructing what is there already. If we are struggling with the uncertainty and the change, we must remind ourselves of the bigger picture – what we are working towards – and remember that the *re*construction phase will come.

So why do we need to deconstruct what's there? Because even where it may be *equal*, it is not *equitable*. Not every voice can be heard right now, and one of the voices that is missing, or at least obscured, is the voice of those who have SEND, together with the voices of their families. It is not for someone who has never experienced being neurodivergent to tell our neurodivergent people how they experience the world, and therefore judge what is right for them. We need to make the space to hear these voices – my children's voices, and my voice, and those of my family, so they can be taken into account to positively expand my children's experience of life and education – this is equity. If we care, then it is also our job to facilitate these voices being heard, and not rely on these voices being able to clearly speak as part of the status quo. Some struggle to find words, some will never have words, some speak other languages, some make art instead of verbalizing, and some speak with actions and behaviours. It is for those who can hear – those who care – to find a route in for these different voices.

The same goes for us as parents and carers tunnelling one way to raise the voices and tunnelling the other to reach our children. Finding the route into our child is one of the wonders of being a parent. For those who parent children with additional needs, we are challenged to reach deep into ourselves to find resources and capacity we never knew we had.

Who are my children?

Let me introduce you to my children. My children have a huge number of intersections in their identities, so I will try to outline who they are here, and tackle more of the detail in each area as I move through the book.

Here I'd like to offer a word of caution: to help readers keep my children clear in their minds, I have given each a pseudonym (Ch1, Ch2, Ch3, Ch4) and provided a bullet-point list of identity words that describe each individual. However, children are not their labels. They are wonderfully complex and are so much more than the sum total of all their descriptors – or their behaviours, for that matter. My children can no more be reduced to a bullet-point list in reality than any other human on the planet.

Child 1

- Dual heritage – Black West Indian and white English
- Dyspraxia
- ADHD
- Non-binary
- Queer
- Fully mainstream schooling

Ch1 was born in 1994, eight years after my husband and I met and six years into our marriage. We were not people who desperately wanted children; we were loving our lives together without them. I think we were also concerned that because our marriage really worked, perhaps a child may change that dynamic, and we wanted to protect the "us" that we had found and created.

By 1994 we were having regular conversations about having a child and imagining what life might look like when our "us" was added to. We tentatively decided we would try … and bingo, I became pregnant in the first month! We were earnest "about-to-be" parents, reading up on parenting and increasing our skills. Most parents (like teachers) have an ideology about how they will nurture their children. It is usually made up from experience of how they were parented: seeing their own parents as an example of how to do it or, conversely, how not to do it. My husband David and I, in those nine months, talked about the nuts and bolts of how we wanted to parent.

Later that year, Ch1 was born. Assigned female at birth (AFAB),[2] we were in absolute awe of this little baby! As with all first-born children, when Ch1 was born they became the baseline in my mind for how a child should be. They talked and walked ahead of their targets. They were chatty, funny, engaging, and very curious. Their entire world seemed to be processed through their mouth. Everything they could fit into their mouth went into their mouth. They would bounce and wave their arms to music and try to sing along. They made eye contact and cuddled everyone. I only realized there may be challenges when they started school. Often, when I went to collect them from school, the teacher would beckon me over for a quick teacher/parent chat. My child was a little too playful and distracted and found it hard to sit still.

By the time they were in Years 2–3 (aged 6–7) I was told this child was rebellious, intentionally inattentive, too loud, and lazy. This is where things can become super-nuanced. If Ch1 had been a blonde, white girl, would the first port of call have been to get the educational psychologist involved to get an assessment? My child is mixed race (white and Afro-Caribbean) and when I think of the language that was used by the school back then, I now realize it could well have been the language of tropes. Lazy, loud, and rebellious are all too familiar terms when it comes to the assessment of our Black and mixed-race children.

Recent studies in the United Kingdom showed Black Caribbean and mixed white and Black Caribbean pupils were noted as being over-represented in the Social, Emotional, and Mental Health (SEMH) area, yet under-represented in the SEN area (Strand and Lindorff, 2021).

This assessment – or even judgement – of my child seemed to be far removed from the child I had at home, who was generally compliant, loved to read, and interacted well, especially with adults. A child's identity is influenced by many factors, but this "naughty" label became problematic – because my child began to believe it.

Today Ch1 has a very strong sense of true north: they are a truth-seeker with incredible gut instincts. If at a young age a child is told the good they possess is bad, this can play havoc with their self-knowledge and the development of their identity. The outside world is in contradiction to the "felt space" in the gut. As a child, who do you believe? The adults are the people who possess the knowledge, so they must be right.

Sadly, as parents, we didn't help this. Having been brought up to respect and trust the school system, on too many occasions we went to town on our child, chastising them for their lack of attention, withholding treats in order to get them to do what the school wanted. Too often we sided with the school, leaving our child supporter-less.

As one would expect, our child began to see themselves as one of the bad kids, so they spent their time with those children who displayed more challenging behaviours. Time and time again, we would be at the school being told our child had been close to something when things went wrong. They were never really the perpetrator, but they were always the bystander. That's clearly where they felt they fitted.

The other challenge was that their reading age was super-advanced but their writing was really behind. They were full of stories, colourful adventures with exuberant, complicated plots. The speed at which their brain would dream up these ideas was supersonic, yet the speed at which they wrote them was snail-paced. They were left-handed and held their pen hard to the page. Homework became a painstaking battle of wills with most of the time being taken up disciplining them; back in the days when we used the naughty step, they pretty much lived on it!

As Ch1 progressed through the school, they had a very good teacher in Year 4. He took me to one side and explained that my child had problems writing their alphabet even though they had an amazing vocabulary and reading skills. He asked if I would concentrate any homework on trying to get them to write their letters. I began by asking Ch1 to write the first few letters. They could manage a, c, e, h, i, and so on … but there were gaps. Anything with a tail was a challenge. I realized they were missing almost half of the letters. And so the painstaking task began to work on simply forming the letters on the page. This was, of course, totally frustrating for Ch1, as they were reading books aimed at 12-year-olds at the age of eight. Recognizing words was easy; *writing* them was a problem.

They began to struggle with confidence. The inability to write well added an extra layer of disconnection to learning, and now they were even more easily distracted. Gazing out the window, they would be called to attention. Clicking their pen, they would be told to be quiet. This lack of clicking the pen meant they would turn their head back to the window. In utter frustration, the teacher would accuse them of wilful disobedience, and they would be called to the front of the class or, worse, sent out of the class.

Throughout this period, however, they continued to prosper at home, playing musical instruments, singing, songwriting, and engaging in many creative pursuits. And thankfully, when Ch1 turned 10, something happened to disrupt the cycle: they gained a professional role in a television drama. This necessitated time away from school for rehearsals and filming, and they instead received their education through on-set tutors, as rules for child actors dictate. Amazingly, when away from school, Ch1 excelled in their education, and was praised for their speedy learning and ability to take direction. When they returned to school for their final year of primary school, they were like a different child. Away from the continual pressure and feelings of failure, they had become confident. In being told they were good at something, their new confidence grew, and with it their ability also grew, across all subjects.

Ch1 was diagnosed with dyspraxia at the age of 11, and AD(H)D at the age of 18. This late diagnosis was a relief to our child, but also very difficult. By the age of 18, they had experienced years of school judgement. They were demoralized, traumatized, and lacking in academic self-belief. The very institution that was meant to prepare them for life had instead disassembled them, mocking their enthusiastic curiosity and judging their difference as defiance.

No one thanks you for a late diagnosis. I have never met a person who wishes they had been diagnosed later. A diagnosis is the doorway to the discovery of that part of you that is outside of the box. There may be parts of the process that demand a rethink of who we are and where we fit in the world. Negative labels can be a heavy weight to bear, of course, but this is largely because the internet gives very negative views on neurological conditions. The truth is that there will also be explanations, revelations, and wonderful, positive attributes that exist because of this neuro-diversity.

Ch1 used the benefit of having intense interests to begin a journey of self-discovery through the lens of their AD(H)D. Suddenly things began to fall into place, frustrations were explained, anxieties more keenly understood. They recognized their ability for fantastic thoughts, yet the struggle they encountered trying to order those thoughts. Suddenly things began to make sense. Not only this, but they began to put things in place in order to assist themselves in the areas where they were struggling – really simple solutions like sending voice notes when they found it hard to reply to people's messages, journaling their thinking, meditation, and most importantly asking for help. When in conflict, they began to slow down the conversation in order to be able to think, taking time out to process thoughts and feelings. Over time, life has become so much easier.

Child 2

- Dual heritage – Black West Indian and white English
- Autistic
- Dyscalculic
- Non-binary masculine
- Queer
- Fully mainstream schooling, with work undertaken at home

Born in 2001, our second child was the hidden child. Assigned female at birth, they were later to realize the correct pronouns to describe them are "he" or "they". Ch2 was quiet and self-contained, and in our words would be described as "in their own world". They would line their toys up, draw pictures all over their walls, and dance to their own rhythm, quite literally … they could beatbox before they could talk. Visitors would say that this child could see "into them"; Ch2 could be unnerving in their habit of observing things and people around them. This part of them has never left, but the way we talk about it has changed: as an adult, we would say that they are unbelievably insightful about others' feelings. They would later be diagnosed as being autistic. The sensory overload that many autistic people experience includes, for this child, the emotions of other people. Imagine walking into a room and feeling everyone's emotions without being able to stop it: this is what Ch2 experiences.

Where Ch1 had jumped up for cuddles and run up for nestling into us, Ch2 was quite the opposite. They would come into our bed in the morning, lie next to me and wait. Instinctively, I knew I needed to create another way into my child's world. It never occurred to me that they might be lacking in anything; I just knew that this child had a different way of communicating and so I unconsciously used my parallel skills to enter the relationship. I would lay my hand on the pillow and tell Ch2 I was going to sleep but Mr Hand would like to chat. This would unlock a super-imaginative and loquacious conversation with my hand. In contrast to the quiet child lying next to me, their parent, they would be giggling, sharing, disclosing, hugging, and kissing my hand. Bit by bit, Ch2 would reverse into me as they talked to my hand, nestled and secure. I found the whole experience delightful and every bit as intimate as the hugs from my first child.

Again, it was school that changed our thinking about our child. At school, Ch2 was highly anxious, felt unheard, and found schoolgirl friendships far too complicated and risky. On constant high alert, they would hold everything together at school, and the minute school was over they would melt down at home. Suddenly, they could only sit at a certain part of the dining table, foods must not touch, and various fears and phobias arose.

Looking back, I think we normalized these changes. It wasn't until a few years later, when our third child was born, that things became a little clearer for me.

Child 3

- Dual heritage – Black West Indian and white English
- Autistic
- ADHD
- Non-binary: demi-girl[3]
- Lesbian
- Mainstream plus specialist autism school

"Do you think she may be deaf?"

This is just one of countless opening lines to conversations my husband David and I began having when Ch3 (assigned female at birth, pronouns she/they, born in 2006) turned two. She wouldn't answer us, respond very much, or turn her head when called. Yet at other times she would be giggly, engaging, and curious, and appeared to hear perfectly.

That spring, we decided to visit friends in Atlanta in the United States, and coming through the airport were stuck on a shuttle train with very high-pitched white noise. Ch3 put her hands to her ears and began to scream. The screaming went on way after the noise had stopped, and even when the screaming stopped her hands remained on her ears.

Over the coming weeks, Ch3 would hold her hands to her ears on and off all day. If there was a loud bang, the extractor fan buzzing, the kettle boiling, and eventually even the low hum of the fridge – hands to ears in clear discomfort. She certainly didn't have a hearing problem! Venturing out became tricky as we were potty training, and if we visited a public toilet the sound of someone using the hand-dryer would have her running from the cubicle mid-flow. The world through Ch3's eyes suddenly looked fraught with danger, and she experienced fearful reactions to everything around her.

Ch3 was also a bit quirky. We love quirky in our house, so we celebrated her desire to wear every outfit off one shoulder; we delighted in her obsession to do up and undo buttons (although this was not so good with those of complete strangers); and we thought it adorable when she referred to herself in the third person.

The noise issue was a problem, though, so I decided to take her to see our local health visitor. This lady had been in the profession for many years and was about to retire. Ch3, in her usual off-the-shoulder attire, took one look at the health visitor's cardigan and began a quest to undo and do up her buttons. The health visitor observed Ch3 for about five minutes and said, "I think she may be autistic." Ch3 was referred for an autism assessment.

This was a key moment where things could have gone one of two ways. Had that health visitor not been so knowledgeable and attentive, Ch3 would have started nursery with everyone none the wiser about what was going on. Starting the diagnostic process later could have been very detrimental to Ch3's experience of school and her young mental health. I am forever grateful for that health visitor's expertise and professionalism in pushing for the assessment. In fact, it gave me great delight years later when I became the president of the Community Practitioners and Health Visitors Union (CPHVA), to be able to give something back.

While waiting for the assessment, David and I began to read about autism and alarm bells began ringing for Ch3's older sibling, Ch2. Ch2 was then seven years old. Those early memories of them lining up toys and only eating certain foods that must not touch each other came flooding back. At school they were terrified of black and white photographs, or anything old. They were outstanding at art and dance and all things creative. They found it hard to navigate school, friendships were complicated, they were bullied, and they felt teachers didn't like them. Years later, Ch2 would describe this as "feeling like an alien".

Ch2 hit their school grades, though, and ticked all the right boxes for "school normal". We were told they were "fine", yet every school day was a living hell.

Neither of these children identifies as female any more, but I do want to take a moment to talk about the fact that autism in girls or those assigned female at birth often doesn't get picked up. There are many shades of autism, but one undisputable fact is that girls often fly under the radar. The child may be very outgoing, sociable, make eye contact, or have an outstanding vocabulary, but beneath the surface could be struggling to understand or comprehend the world around them. They may have overwhelming sensory issues and a rigid, very concrete way of understanding what is being said. This social communication issue may leave the child feeling as if they are in a war zone at school, with teachers shouting, demands not understood and therefore felt as threatening, and threats of detention or punishment. Friendships are confusing, baffling, bewildering, painful. Feelings of not fitting in and an alarming, ever-growing sense of failure eventually lead to self-hatred. Daily meltdowns at home lead to school refusal, and eventually result in complete shutdown and/or mental breakdown. By the age of nine, our beautiful Ch2 was asking to die, and unfortunately it was only at this point that we were taken seriously. Maybe this was autism but not as we knew it?

But why should this be the case? The simplest reason is that until recently it was believed that autism was a male condition, and most of the research had been done on males, or those assigned male at birth. So what does this mean for girls? We know less about how autism presents in girls, and we can't spot it as easily as we might in a little boy. Added to this, teachers are given very little SEND training generally, let alone specific autism training. Then there is the commonly held trope of all autistic people making no eye contact and selecting to be mute but having a savant skill – it's problematic. If these are the only traits people are looking for, how are girls ever going to get the help they need? Diagnosed males used to outnumber females ten to one. That figure currently stands at three to one, but is still suspected to be skewed (National Autistic Society, 2021).

David and I decided to take both Ch2 and Ch3 for a private assessment, and one afternoon in the summer of 2008 we were told that both children were autistic. Many parents talk about the grief they feel when their child is diagnosed with autism. It is important to be authentic and allow oneself to process what it truly means to be autistic or to have an autistic child/sibling/ student. Unfortunately, the internet can be a negative place to research autism. For many years, autistic voices have been absent in discussions and comments about autism. We have heard from the professionals and we have heard from the parents, who have almost entirely spoken about the challenges without balance and without hope. This has meant that any newcomer is plunged into relentless negativity.

To be honest, David and I didn't grieve at all. Our children were the same delightful children after someone diagnosed them as they had been hours before. David and I have ourselves always felt different; indeed, we celebrate difference in our family. Our job as vocal coaches is about seeking those artists who are different

– difference is an advantage in our world. Our grief came later, with the fight to have our children's needs met at school and in healthcare. Academic research shows that the mothers of autistic children experience "combat-like" levels of stress (Diament, 2009). But it is also most often assumed that the source of the stress is the child themselves, when most parents would say it is fighting the system that causes the most harm.

For those parents who have very clear expectations for their children, and who then feel that those expectations are gone, there may be a necessary period of time to grieve. Part of that process is actually looking at why we feel that we have to all grow up to be the same, and why culturally we have a particular results-based model for adulthood and life.

If you are a professional meeting parent(s) who have just been told that their child is autistic, they may well be trying to process what this means. The greatest thing these parents need is not your knowledge or your pity, but your empathy. Working through anything is not always neat and tidy, so please, allow them to be angry, confused, and emotionally wrung out.

Child 4

- Dual heritage – Black African and white English
- Dyspraxia
- ADHD
- Attachment Disorder
- Mainstream school and Pupil Referral Unit

And so to our fourth child, who was born in 2009 and joined our family in 2011. I'm sure some people wondered why, when we already had children who were different, we would then choose to adopt another child. We have often been asked this question. We would say the biggest challenges for us have been in accessing health and navigating the education system. The children themselves are great. The issues we find that challenge us as parents are usually their mental health issues, most of which come from being traumatized by school, not from their actual difference. Of course, some of the answer is that we did not yet know some of the difficulties and challenges our family would face. Most of the mental health issues my children have faced became more difficult as they entered into secondary school at the age of 11, and our youngest two children – our autistic children – were ten and nearly four at the point when we adopted.

But that's not the whole answer to the question of why we chose to adopt Ch4. Our home is a bustling, busy, person-centred place, where people share and find fellow travellers. In 2011, we had been married for 23 years. Our lives had expanded over the years and the thought of another addition to our family felt right. We didn't go out looking to adopt: our friend, who was a foster carer, came to us and asked whether we would consider adopting a little boy she was caring for. He was about to turn two, he was of dual heritage, and he was a boy. These three details would mean he would be less likely to be picked up for adoption in the United Kingdom. On paper, he fitted with our family and looked like a family member. Our children all agreed that they wanted to have a new family member … and so we embarked on the journey to welcome this little boy into our family.

In adoption training, we were taught about attachment, and told that adoption was a lifelong issue for an adoptee. We found that really hard to accept at the time; I think we felt that "love wins", and so there would be a natural bonding and healing process, and if we could just love him enough, change would occur over a few years. The lesson we have had to learn as family is that it is not our job to change people; it is our job to sit alongside in the muck and the mire, and *listen* with all our hearts.

Ch4 had gone into foster care at the age of four months, and remained there until he came to us at the age of two. It is not our place to tell his early life story, but suffice to say that in the United Kingdom, there is usually good reason for children to be placed into care. Ch4 was super-connected to his foster carer, so adoption for him was like a critical break in his heart. He grieved every day, standing by the window waiting for her return. He yearned for his old home and struggled to accept that we were his "forever family".

In truth, he bonded well with my husband, David. David is Black, and a man, and was therefore outside Ch4's prior experience. It was me he struggled with. It was as though I had kidnapped him; he absolutely *hated* me. He would lavish love onto David and reject me constantly. Adoption can be hard. It can test you to your very core. It is so important to remain adult and remain consistent. On reflection, and over the years, I think I have managed this, but I can tell you it has not been without a lot of self-talk, and many times I have felt like giving up on the whole thing (not on Ch4 – I have never contemplated giving up on him). Like many adoptees, Ch4 did not have the very basic structures for emotional and mental security. The backdrop to the parent–child relationship is so very different from that of a birth child. As a mother, I could not pour love where there was no capacity. I had to wait for the capacity to open up; I had to earn the capacity and hold onto my love until such a time as it would be ready to be received.

Ch4 spent months grieving. He found it hard to make decisions about anything. He feared making choices about everyday tasks such as what cereal he would eat for breakfast, or what toy he should play with. Not happy for others to make those choices for him, he was in constant fight or flight mode. If he made a choice and then deemed the decision a wrong one, he would go and hide, defaulting into shame, and unable to move from the position either geographically or emotionally. I would just sit further away in the room and try to hold the space, but for years I was ignored. If Ch4 hurt himself, he would hide, hating to show vulnerability, and if we tried to help him he would lash out in anger at us. It's very hard when you are both the problem and the solution. This continued into nursery and then school, which is when everything escalated.

With the structure and expectation of school, Ch4 couldn't cope at all. He lashed out, hitting both children and teachers, and causing serious harm to the adults. He was isolated and assigned a teaching assistant (TA), and spent about two years alone with the TA in the school gym, away from others in case he caused harm. He would also hit me at home, punching me full in the face, knocking me to the floor. School could not manage the behaviour and eventually Ch4 was moved to another school. He was placed in what is known as a Pupil Referral Unit (PRU) attached to a large hospital, where expertise could be found.

We felt completely under-equipped, so one of the first things we did was to have some trauma therapy. Understanding trauma and its impact on the body and mind was a huge revelation and this helped us to understand both our child and our own responses to what was happening. I fully understood that if the body keeps score, and I was holding all my pain inside me, then this was not going to be healthy for me going forward. Seeking help was the best thing we could have done, as we could bounce ideas off someone outside of the situation. I have always been desperate to learn and, after a while, desperate to find people who know more than I do. Experts give me hope, because when it comes to my children, my impetus and driving desire cannot be "change them!" – I never want to make my children feel like I do not love them exactly as they are and for who they are. If a situation between my children and I is not working, the acceptable solution is only ever "change me!"

Looking back at that time, I would say this was the most difficult time for David and me in our parenting journey. We were so ill-equipped and under-prepared, and on totally different pages. We began our parenting journey with very clear ideas about how we would parent, and we both agreed we would be quite strict, playful, disciplined, and boundaried. David pulled into the original plan, which clearly wasn't working for me.

We were in total disagreement, and at this point our parenting was no longer working for any of our children … or either of us, for that matter. The professionals really helped. They explained that with these children, "regular" parenting would not work. We had to deconstruct our learning and work out how to be what we needed to be for *these particular children*, and not even expect to parent all four the same way. Every child needed a bespoke methodology. This was super-parenting; this was shape-shifter parenting. It would take everything we had within us to evolve. It would mean digging deep, communicating even more, and growing into being the parents we needed to be.

Alongside the trauma therapy, we also learned about non-violent resistance (NVR). NVR takes the principles of political resistance used by Martin Luther King, Mahatma Gandhi and Nelson Mandela and transforms them into a parenting format. I will go into greater detail about this later in this book, but NVR changed us and put us on the same page as one another. It worked very well for Ch4, and he stopped being violent towards me. Now he is a joy to be around. He is chatty, sweet, friendly, loving, kind, helpful, generous, funny, and a whole list of good stuff. Like his siblings, though, school has been another matter, and continues to be a big problem to this day. The school in which he was most recently enrolled is amazing, but for some reason school exacerbates the trauma he feels. Most of the time he is the same delightful child as he is at home, but he finds it hard to self-regulate and presents with some very challenging behaviours. Absconding, violence, damage to property, injuries to adults … the challenging behaviours continue. The police are called to the school regularly, and we are called upon to work even more closely with one another.

How we see children

So, as you can see, our children are a whole amazing mix. It would be a wonderful world if every child, or even every person, could be known just as they are – if every identity word perfectly captured the truth of each experience; if everyone understood the same things about what it means to be a woman, or autistic, or Black. Of course, this is not the case, and one of the most significant issues for both parents and professionals is that when we view a child, we can only ever view them through the prism of our own experience. This means that in order to work towards greater understanding of each other – and especially of the children in our care – we need to be constantly questioning and interrogating our own assumptions. A child may present with "challenging behaviours", for example … but who are they challenging to? When we understand that that child is in constant fight-or-flight mode, we may understand why they are alternately trying to escape and hitting out. An "under-the-radar" autistic girl may simply appear totally comfortable, if a bit shy. But if we understand how this child may be experiencing the world – perhaps as a bewildering cacophony of mysterious expectations and an alien landscape – then we start to truly see this child. Of course, every child is completely unique with their own way of experiencing the world, but it is our job to pick up the trail of breadcrumbs they are leaving in their wake and to remain curious about what we notice. Our assumptions and projections can trip us up.

Belonging

Every child matters and every story needs to be included. As for me, partly because of who my children are, I have made it my life's aim to jump between stories, to become a bridge to different worlds. Perhaps this is in order to make sense of those different worlds myself, but ultimately I want to bring people together. More often than not, in the heart of people is a deep desire to be known and to belong. If our children are constantly made to feel they don't belong, this impacts their identity and shapes who they become. People with SEN should not have to justify their existence; they need to be accepted as equal and included in the belonging – not tolerated, sidelined, or marginalized, but *fully belonging*.

Knowledge and the gift of teaching

Growing in knowledge is one of the most fantastic things in life, especially when it leads to applied knowledge. Those with the gift of passing on knowledge are to be treasured. It is a skill, and it has a purpose. I have a career in coaching and I know that what I do goes way beyond the details and techniques I impart. Teaching and learning involve creativity and play. We see how one piece of information links to another, and suddenly science, history, philosophy, art, and culture all interact. They create a picture for the learner and a foundation for their developing worldview. In this world of learning, we are unlocking something magical.

Taking measurements

We also live in a world obsessed with evidence-gathering, and the system we have created measures our academic learning through the medium of exams. There are limitations with using exams as a metric: it may not measure the application of what we have learned, it may not measure its cross interactions with other subjects, it may not judge the creative force within us, or our strengths or our gifts; but it will measure how much of the academic learning we are able to remember, and this impacts how teachers teach.

So, there are two things at play here: an over-emphasis on academic learning, and examinations to test academic retention. Academic achievement has been given a supreme pedestal: as a society, we have worshipped it and weaponized it. We have used it to create a narrative that tells children this is all they are worth. In turn, we have told teachers that if they do not hit targets, they also lack worth. I have seen this with all four of my children: their individual struggle to find out who they are and where their worth lies, when the message they are receiving from school is that their gifts are not valued and their so-called "failures" define them. I have also seen how some of their teachers struggle to know how to do what they want to do and are supposed to do – teach – when the system they have to work within is not one that meets my children where they are. Something has to change.

Creativity in learning

There has long been an argument between those who believe school should focus on the STEM subjects (Science, Technology, Engineering, and Maths) and those who believe in STEAM (Science, Technology, Engineering, Arts, and Maths). Ch2 is highly gifted as an artist and sportsperson. They constantly struggled to find any inner confidence at school; they felt invisible, unnoticed by a school system and teachers who valued things they did not find easy, and did not value the things that they excelled at. Two incidents illustrate the negative impact that school had on their life through this narrow focus on STEM subjects.

By the age of 11, Ch2 was terrified of going up into "big school", having already learned from the last few years that school did not value their skills or personality. As their parent, I was thinking of ways to try and ease their path in, and create an early opportunity for success – I had hopes that a new school would provide something of a fresh start. I noticed that the new school had a "gifted and talented" register – perhaps this could be something to forge a positive connection between Ch2 and their new school? Ch2 had just won the World Taekwondo Championships, so I approached the school to ask whether my child's achievements could be recognized with a "gifted and talented" status. However, I was quickly disappointed:

> "Sorry, it's only for students who are outstanding in English, Maths or Science."

That's not even STEM. To the school, sport was largely an extracurricular activity, and excellence in sport didn't count as "gifted" or "talented". It's probable that if my child had won Young Musician of the Year, the response would have been the same. What a missed opportunity to encourage a child to engage in the community of a new school.

Then, in that same school a few years later, Ch2 was present when in an assembly for Year 11's Careers Day, a slide was put up in front of all the children present. It was a montage photograph of different TV programmes – all shows or scenes that might be held up as aspirational by young people who value pop culture. The opening line of the head teacher's speech was:

> "None of you are going to do this."

In a criticism both of many young people's values and of modern life, the head could not see any value in the arts. Instead of using the opportunity to inspire young people, to promote ambition and aspiration, the choice was made to squash and crush. My child got up and walked out – an action that only added to the reputation of being "difficult" that children with SEN can attract, but one I understand. And the action was justified, not only in that moment but later: one year after that assembly, they were nominated as Best Newcomer in a National TV Drama category that has set them on a career pathway in the arts, proving that the head's speech was categorically wrong. Imagine how much easier that career path might have been to develop had Ch2 experienced encouragement and cultivation – had their voice been heard and valued in their own education.

Incidentally, not only have they started a career of their choosing, but they have also paid a lot of tax into the government's coffers, and from a much younger age than many who would follow a more academic path. From an economic point of view, they are "viable", despite everything they were told by society – and school – growing up. It appears that those who create policy and get to decide what the emphasis will be have forgotten the power and economic importance of the arts.

Creativity is fundamental to who we are as humans. That is not to say we are all artists, but in some way all of us have the power to create. The best scientists will be those who can think outside of the box – the creative thinkers. Those who build companies and become successful in business would be nothing without creativity. Creativity is not an after-school club; it is essential to our continuing existence.

Local and national governance

When we look at the aims of local government, what do we find?

Our aim is to remove barriers to learning, ensure that children and young people will feel that their achievements are valued, that they are happy and enjoy school, lead healthy lifestyles, feel safe in their learning environments and are appropriately supported in order to achieve their full potential.

(Dudley SEND Strategic Launch, 2021)

Sometimes we find good work being done at the local level. Certainly, the aims are good – as a parent and advocate, I can find nothing in the above aim that's not to like. However, we also know the system is under incredible strain, both financially and in the way our professional services are led. From my point of view, many professionals appear to be doing the work of three people. They are exhausted, and of course this leads to sickness and extended absence, which in turn leads to delays in parents accessing help, ultimately leading to the child not coping in school.

Health and education

It is my absolute belief that health, social care, and education should have a joint department, working together to provide a bedrock of good mental health and creating lifelong learners. In July 2021, I posted a tweet, having read a quote from our then Minister of State for Mental Health, Suicide Prevention and Patient Safety, The Rt Hon Nadine Dorries MP. At an All-Party Parliamentary Meeting, Dorries had said, "CAMHS is well-resourced and robust." I simply added to the quote, "Has anyone got anything to say about this? What's your experience?".

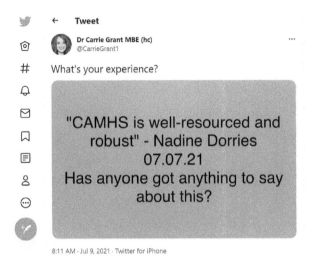

Figure 2 Tweet from @CarrieGrant1, 9 July 2021

The tweet, with its 3.5 million impressions (i.e. the total number of times a tweet is seen, including search results and shares), trended for two days. Reading the responses to that tweet is heartbreaking. It is full of stories of real-life people whose children are being seriously let down. It is also full of comments from teachers, therapists, and GPs. Notably, not one comment I saw was in agreement with the Minister's original assessment of CAMHS. The saddest part was reading the number of comments from adults whose lives have been upturned by the lack of care and support at health level when they were younger. Health cannot be separated from education: one influences the other, they go hand in hand.

In 2017, I hosted the NHS England Conference, where Director for Mental Health Clare Murdoch talked about the "Five-Year Forward View for Mental Health". At the time, Murdoch shared that only 25 per cent of referrals to CAMHS led to an appointment. She promised this would change, and it has. We are currently four years on from that promise, and the figures are even worse.[4] Young Minds UK's 2019 report shows that CAMHS only accounts for 0.7 per cent of NHS spending, and only 6.4 per cent of mental health spending (Young Minds, 2019). When you consider that 50 per cent of mental health issues are established by the age of 14 (Kessler et al., 2005), it doesn't paint a pretty picture. This bears repeating: although the evidence suggests that half of all mental health problems begin before the age of 15, we are spending more than 93 per cent of all available mental health funds on things other than fostering healthy minds and treating mental health problems in our young people and children.

As a result of the trending tweet, I was asked to write an article for *Special Needs Jungle*. The article, entitled "Dying to Be Seen" (Grant, 2021), challenges us all to think about the damage that is done when there are delays in access to care. If a child cannot access mental health support when they are self-harming or have suicidal ideation because they do not meet the threshold, something has gone seriously wrong. The trending tweet and following article were written just days after I had intervened in my child's latest suicide attempt – a few months after the previous suicide attempt, when we had been promised help from CAMHS.

And so again we come back to the point that health and education are inextricably linked. More often than not, once a child is in this spiralling position, it is likely that they will begin to refuse to go to school. If the school cannot meet the needs of the child – which initially may have entailed fairly minor adjustments – then it is inevitable that it will tell parents it cannot meet the needs of the child once those needs increase. There are many children in the United Kingdom who have been off-rolled, excluded, or expelled in this way and left without school. Nationally, 2017 figures indicate a very high rate of exits from schools: as many as one in 10 pupils (10.1%) in the 2017 cohort experienced exits at some point during their time at secondary school that cannot be accounted for (Hutchinson and Crenna-Jennings, 2019).

The system is so slow it can take years for things to catch up, if they do so at all, and in the meantime parents become full-time carers, therapists, and educators. The economic impact has never been measured, but you can imagine.

Why are we losing teachers?

In addition to the resourcing challenges faced by CAMHS and other health and social care services, the education system in the United Kingdom is just as pressed. The teaching sector is trying to work out why they are losing so many people in the profession – it's obviously something they're keen to change. But from my perspective, I don't know if we have to look too hard to find the answer. A 2021 survey from the National Education Union of 10,000+ school and college staff reported that:

- 70% said the workload had increased over past year, with almost all respondents (95%) reporting they were worried about the impact on their wellbeing;
- 35% of total respondents reported that they would definitely no longer be working in education in five years' time;
- 66% said the status of the profession had got worse, with government blamed for failing to listen to or value them.

When asked why, those who indicated that they would no longer be working in education, either in two or five years' time, said the most common reason was that the education profession was not valued or trusted by government/media (53%), closely followed by workload (51%), then accountability (34%), and pay (24%) (National Education Union, 2021).

It is really important when we question a teacher's motivation and drive to also understand the pressure they face from systemic issues.

Teaching is a vocation

Without putting these issues aside, how do we rediscover the vocational status of teaching? How do we provide a landscape where teachers are encouraged to be inspirational, positive, and forward thinking? Despite the pressure and struggle faced by many schools, I do believe there is some great work being done out there – I have witnessed it. But largely it's still down to those one-off teachers who happen to have a natural instinct towards inclusion and diversity and who are willing to embrace change.

When we look at the landscape, it can make us want to give up. Why bother? It can feel like it's too difficult to know where to begin to effect change. Parents have no choice but to keep going. We need every ally we can find. We need you to care. We need your compassion, we need your listening ear, we need you to use your ability and status to make sure every child matters, every child is considered and every child is given whatever is needed in order to reach their full potential.

We need great leaders.

Learning objective: Leadership in all its forms

To think about leadership in the widest sense and in all its forms. To consider what it might mean to be a leader in your own context, and what it might mean to inspire leadership in others.

2
Leadership

What does great leadership look like? For the past 23 years, I have worked as a leadership coach with thousands of people across a whole range of companies, from health services to government bodies, from coffee companies to road builders, from supermarket chains to betting shops.

Hero leader

As the twentieth century "doff your cap" days have begun to fade, the leadership arena now talks about collaboration and team building. There is a massive shift occurring. Up until the last 20 years, a leader was a white, university-trained man in his forties or fifties. This man had a charismatic character, was a super-engaging public speaker, and led by stealth through the sheer weight of his brilliant personality. He was also expected to know everything. Not knowing something would have been perceived as weakness. Collaboration would have been regarded as indecision or an over-reliance on others, and an inability to personally own the issue. We can call this leadership type the "hero-leader" – someone who thinks they have to be a superhero in order to lead effectively.

For the first five years of training leaders, we didn't meet one leader who didn't have this profile. As a white woman and Black man brought into train these leaders, we were an anomaly. To begin with, we didn't understand why we were there. Not only were we different both in terms of gender and race, but we were also artists, the touchy-feely people who think about how the space in the room is being held, asking who's controlling the temperature, and working out how we influence the space – definitely not the "know-everything" type of leader I've just described. Over time, though, we came to realize that the very reason we had been brought in was to challenge the status quo. It was to encourage these leaders to bring their humanity, their vulnerability, their discomfort, and their disclosure into the room.

Believe it or not, we used singing to achieve our goals. Can you imagine? It was painful for them, and a wonderful leveller, which eventually led to unity and connection in the room. We helped them to sit with discomfort and invited them to trust us *unusual* people in the process. We saw transformation. Over the past two decades, we have seen a new type of leader emerging. This leader is both a seer (see-er) and a coach. This leader can admit that there are things they don't know, and can look to other members of the team to find those skills and giftings. The seer/coach leader's job is to use their seeing skills to look at a team member without judgement, and to work out and identify what gifts and skills are within that person – even when they may not know it themselves yet. The coach part then draws the gifts and skills to the surface. This leader will also inevitably see the areas of weakness and help the person to be aware of how those weaknesses may mitigate against the strengths. The message we try to demonstrate through our coaching is that getting to call the shots does not mean we lose our humanity: all can work together to find equality and respect. An effective team is not about a group of people vying for pole position; it is about each person understanding their unique strengths, where they fit and what they bring to the group DNA.

The point is this: if this kind of human and humane leadership is happening in school, there is a greater likelihood that this attitude of inclusion and acceptance will filter through to the classroom and community beyond.

Nowadays, there are many ways of doing leadership. The authentic leader brings themselves into the room, loud or shy, serious or funny, sociable or unsociable, practical or cerebral, or any combination of attributes. The good news to new leaders is this: You are enough.

Like likes like; different is a threat

All leadership will inevitably lead to legacy – good or bad. The legacy of the hero-leader is duplication: find someone just like me and pass it on. It doesn't take a genius to see that this approach can only lead to a total lack of inclusion. We only do business with, and pass leadership on to, people who look like us, sound like us, and think like us; it's what we've always done and it works a treat. Sound familiar? We are back to the one empirical story where everyone knows their script (except, of course, we know that not everyone does). Anyone who wants to switch this scene up is accused of being "woke" – a word that, when used with this disparaging overtone, means over-considerate to the margins, or pandering just to look good.[5] Once we step outside of this very narrow, old hero-leader worldview, the whole world opens up … anything can happen! Who knows the types of people we may interact with? A rich diverse mix of every type of human brings massive potential with all its different ways of seeing the world. The dominant script-writers may feel threatened by the presence of someone a little different taking up just a little bit of the space. This "broadening out" may feel like a threat to their existence. As leadership coaches, we have seen this scene play out.

"We could never work with xyz," we hear, usually followed by a lame excuse and often a trope thrown in for good measure. I won't list them here, but think about the many female tropes we have, how many Black and mixed-race tropes, Asian tropes, neurodivergent tropes, LGBTIQ+ tropes, working-class tropes, Muslim tropes, Jewish tropes … the list goes on. Fortunately, though, not everyone is like this. While the world is looking for reasons not to collaborate, there are a growing number of people who are looking at the extraordinary benefits of a rich and diverse community.

School has a fundamental part to play in this leadership revolution. Education has the opportunity to make the next generation collaborative, inclusive, valued, and ultimately unified. Instead of our children learning from the status quo, we have the chance to teach them a better way, and to model better, more fulfilling and more effective leadership in the place where they are supposed to do their learning.

Mindset

When a teacher enters the classroom, they come with a worldview – we all do. What this worldview is doesn't necessarily matter: in the first instance, the issue is not what you know or don't know; it is more about your level of curiosity and ability to adapt your thinking. It's not about what your mindset is, it's about how *pliable* your mindset is. Are you prepared to stretch out your worldview, or does that feel too overwhelming?

My experience of interactions with school is that there is often a pressure on the professional[6] to know everything. This pressure creates a block to communication. Behind a closed mindset is a fear of showing weakness … again, we are back into old-style, hero-leadership thinking. If only our educators could understand that they don't need to know everything; instead, they need to be authentic and willing to learn. Many parents of SEND children will tell you that the people with whom they have the most issues are not those who know nothing, but those who know very little and insist they know everything – and, more pertinently, that they know more than you as parent.

One of my key memories of my children's primary education was a teacher who called me in for a meeting at the beginning of the first term.

> "I really want to get it right with your child [Ch3], but I've had absolutely no autism training. I have a friend who has had more training and I've been asking them questions and I have also read up on some information online, but I really want to get this right."

These few simple sentences were music to my ears. I wasn't upset that the teacher didn't know everything about working with autistic children; I was in fact overjoyed that they cared enough to ask! We then chatted, and the relationship through that year of Ch3's life was outstanding. The teacher was my child's favourite ever, and they loved teaching my child. This is a great example of that pliable mindset – and also a pretty good example of leadership.

Leading as a parent: Learning to be the "warrior parent"

Leadership is not just for the senior leadership team (SLT) at a school. All teachers are leaders – like Ch3's teacher, who led the way in establishing a healthy relationship based on mutual respect and learning. All parents are leaders too, and all children are learning the early pathway towards leadership as they learn to advocate for themselves.

I don't think I fully realized I had to lead in my child's schooling until things got really hard. The system is not set up for parents to have agency; it's not a common experience for parents to be *invited* into leadership in a school – especially parents of SEN children. The role of parent can be a very reductive one in many ways – for example, I am known as Ch1/2/3/4's mum. I cease to be Carrie – I don't even have a name anymore. Yet, a leader is exactly what I needed to be.

One day in 2013, I had my oldest child starting university, my second child starting secondary school, and my youngest starting nursery. Any one of these would be a big day, even in the school journey of a "typical" child, so with three SEND children embarking on significant milestones and changes, I felt I was fire-fighting in every direction! When I look back now, I think it was at this point that I truly became the parent who would fight for my child.

When my under-the-radar Ch2 turned 11 and the primary school had not really engaged with their needs, I knew it would be a problem going into secondary school. This is a situation where children go from one safe class of 30 to hundreds in a year group, with multiple classrooms and multiple teachers. For Ch2, though, they were stepping from an unsafe place to an even more challenging one – their needs were already going unmet, and the chance of them falling through the cracks in secondary school was huge. To try to head this risk off, I applied for a Statement of Needs (now known as an Education/Health Care Plan, or EHCP) in the last year of primary school, knowing that in secondary school it would become essential. An EHCP is a legal document agreed by the Local Authority, which uses it to commit to a budget, which in turn provides the school with the money required to meet the needs of the child, so that ultimately that child can access learning and remain well.

Like many families, we were turned down on the first attempt, so we had to take it to a tribunal. Again, as many parents also experience when they decide to fight for their child's rights, the Local Authority backed down at the last minute and agreed to the EHCP just before the tribunal hearing date. This was an incredible moment. I naively believed that this EHCP was the golden ticket to my child being provided for, that their experience of school would now change, that this would give them equality with their peers. Little did I know that there was a more sinister agenda at work.

**

Off-rolling: A failure of leadership

In the United Kingdom, schools are driven by exam results. The better the results, the higher the school travels up the league table. Schools are assessed by the Office for Standards in Education (OFSTED) and, until very recently, there were no measurements for how schools performed regarding their SEND cohort. A SEND child under-achieving compared with their peers might bring the average results of the school down, without any recognition that for this child, results that appear to be under-achieving through a "typical" lens might actually represent huge progress when you take the child's whole context into account. This pressure on schools meant that some began to "off-roll" students. Like a constructive dismissal, life for our SEND students in some schools began to be so unbearable that they would end up out of school, and eventually be taken off the register of that school – without the bad press of actually *excluding* that child.

There are thousands of children currently out of school. Some remain on the school register even though they do not attend, while others are taken off the register. Many of these children have no provision, so parents have to leave work to care for their child full-time. The parent/carer is expected to be parent, educator, and therapist. If this situation doesn't make us into parent-leaders, I don't know what will! We are the parents struggling to get EHCPs – which cannot be awarded unless the child is in school – when our children are not in school (but we need the EHCP to get out child back into school). How's that for a catch-22? We are the parents being told that our suicidal child does not meet the threshold for access to care. This is what happens when there is a failure of good leadership.

***

Ch2 refused to go to school. They had the EHCP, but getting the school to actually apply it was another challenge we hadn't expected. I was told that if they made adjustments for Ch2, then they would have to make adjustments for everyone. I argued that my child was autistic and was told none of the other young people were aware of this and they wouldn't disclose. When I tried to email a teacher about Ch2's needs, I was told I was not allowed to make contact with anyone but the one lead person. I tried to report bullying and the first thing I encountered was victim shaming. My child was on suicide watch in hospital, and *still being bullied*, and still nothing was done. When I spoke to the SLT, I was told that for my child, having no friends was to be expected and that they had seen it happen over and over with autistic girls in secondary school. And when I wrote to the one point of contact I was allowed to access, begging for help, someone more senior told them:

> "Now stand well back and watch the fireworks …
> You do not have to reply to all of her emails …"

The person who wrote this email, mistakenly sent it *to* me when it was supposed to be *about* me without my knowledge; they then tried to retrieve the email … but I had already opened it. I think this was one of the lowest points for me: to be treated with such contempt, ignored, and manipulated. I felt powerless and my child was utterly broken. They were asking me to make the changes, asking me to make a way for them – but I could not do it. I could not make school listen, and I could not make a difference. I could not offer my child hope, because there was no hope. I had failed my child.

Effective leaders need community

In response to these overwhelming feelings, I reached out to every supporter I had – anyone who could help me – and in the process I learned what I could fight for. I formed a support group for parents and the young people themselves. If I had no voice, I reasoned, I would have to *find* one. I found one professional who knew the law, and I found one supporter in my Local Authority – they made a way where there was no way and I will be forever grateful to them.

Now, finally, we started to see some adjustments and some support. If Ch2 couldn't make it into school, the TA would make notes for the lessons they had missed. And even greater than this, my Local Authority insisted that the school send the TA to our house, if necessary, to pass on the learning. Unfortunately, the whole process took my child from age 11 until the age of 16 before the full support kicked in – and the best example of full support wasn't actually from school at all, in the end. Ch2 went on to be the first autistic female (as they were presenting at the time; now they identify as non-binary/trans) to star in a UK TV drama.

The company who make the continuing drama in question, Lime Pictures, gave two days' autism training to all the cast and crew. This effectively means a lighting rigger on that soap opera has had more autism training than *any teacher who ever taught Ch2 in their whole school career.* Take a second to let that sink in!

And what difference did it make to have the agreed adjustments made, and Ch2's needs met? It has meant that they have been able to travel to work over 200 miles away every week, learn scripts, stay away from home, and work under pressure – in stark contrast to being unable to even go in for part of a school day. What a difference good leadership makes.

The warrior parent fighting multiple battles

In the midst of Ch2's struggles, things were also looking tricky for our other children. In the final year of primary school, Ch3 found it difficult to self-regulate and stay in class. This led to behaviours that were seen as disruptive – perhaps understandably, unless you understand why they are happening and where they are coming from. For example, they might call over a teacher to look at a book, and when the teacher leant over them to see, they shut the book. On the surface, this is rude, highly irritating and, yes, disruptive. But when you dig a little deeper and realize that Ch3 was craving attention, engagement, and stimulation, but struggled to receive it in the ways other children in the classroom could, it starts to make a little more sense – and the way you should respond to the behaviour starts to look different too. In reality, behaviours like this led to Ch3 being excluded from school every afternoon until they could complete three out of five tasks three mornings in a row. The only trouble was at least two of the tasks they were being asked *not* to do were autistic traits. (And let's not even start with the backwards-ness of assigning a negative task – your task is to *not* do this, instead of a positive, "achieve this" type task.) This inability to shed their autistic traits – such as stimming[7] – in order to meet this checklist led to a crazy cycle of me picking them up from school every day at noon for a month. By being unable to manage these three tasks for three days in a row – a seemingly simple challenge that was actually designed to be impossible – they were set up to fail. The cycle was only broken when Ch2 went back into hospital, and I physically couldn't pick Ch3 up. How could I lead in this situation?

I fully understood that Ch3's behaviours were challenging the mainstream school, so I applied for a secondary placement in a specialist all-girls autism school. By this time it was 2017 and the old Statement of Needs system had been replaced by EHCPs. As part of their transfer to an EHCP, all their reports had to be updated and it was at this point that they were diagnosed as having ADHD as well as being autistic. This extra layer can make things more challenging. As I heard someone say once, "My ADHD brain keeps writing cheques that my autism brain can't cash!"

Eventually, Ch3 got a place in an amazing autism school 90 minutes from where we live … but sadly, even this was not without challenges. At that time, they were questioning their gender and sexuality, and the whole family were supporting them through the changes and experiences they were feeling. Ch3 wore a coat all day at school and a hat all day and night. It was like a security blanket and also a shield from other children, keeping out stares and noise. In the new school, they had to be in uniform, with no coat and no hat. The new school did not bend the rules on this, and as we were trying to work with the school in the hope that it would work for Ch3, we went along with them. We encouraged our child to take off the outer garments. Looking back now, I can see that this must have felt like asking them to enter school stark naked, with no protection.

The new school had some amazing results with their autistic girls (and those assigned female at birth), but perhaps the type of children they drew were those who were under the radar, the shy ones like Ch2, not the blurty, non-masking children like Ch3. Once again, we were in a situation where Ch3's natural behaviours were seen as disruptive, which led to them being put in a room alone with a TA, all day, every day. One day I was flying to Ireland for work and just about to turn my phone onto airplane mode when a whole line of texts appeared:

"HELP"
"PLEASE HELP ME"
"COME AND GET ME"
"I CAN'T TAKE THIS ANYMORE"
"HELP"
"HELP ME"
"PLEASE ANSWER"
"COME AND GET ME"
"PLEASE"

… and I switched my phone off for take-off. I did not feel at the time that I could – or even should – have done anything else. We so badly wanted this new school to be the solution for Ch3. I had not yet admitted to myself that this new environment might be yet another battlefield where I would need to fight for the health and happiness of my child.

Ch3 lasted just a few weeks in the school. Traumatized and alone, they returned home and hid themselves away in their bedroom. The Local Authority sent home-learning TAs to the house, but still Ch3 refused to come downstairs. The message they had received loud and clear was, "You do not fit in this world."

Again, I reflected on what leadership looked like in this instance. How could we all have done things better? Where did it go wrong? When and how could I step in for my child without falling out with the school? How could school leaders set the tone to create the right environment for collaboration? What constitutes a behaviour that challenges? And who is it challenging?

Always moving forward

But in real life, there is often very little time to stop and reflect – any looking back has to be done while continuing to move forward. In our case, school had well and truly come to our home; TAs for both Ch2 and Ch3 would arrive, with David and I hosting and waiting for children to come downstairs and learn. It was to remain like this for three years for Ch3, from the age of 11 to nearly 15. We relied once again on our wonderful Local Authority, who really listened to us. Soon Ch3 had two young, trendy and very relatable TAs, and even a curriculum of sorts, built around their desires. They had dog training, cooking and drama club, piano lessons, and trips out to museums and markets. They also had English, maths, and science work that they completed. Slowly, they began to re-engage. There was very little socialization, so their friendships only really existed online. This is not the best way to do things by a long way – but we were moving forward at least.

My parent-leading was not just growing at childhood education level; it also had to take on leadership at university level. Ch1 had been diagnosed with ADHD the year before going to university. Knowing this, they had built a whole system designed to make sure they didn't fail. Every day, they carried every single study book in their bag so that they would not forget books. They struggle with interoception (the ability to know when your body needs food or the toilet), so would make sure they went to the toilet before lessons to avoid disruptions. However, the geography of buildings is a mystery to them, so having popped to the toilet they would not be able to find where the next class was. Arriving late, they would settle down, taking out all the books, pens, and clothing for that session. In order to stay alert, they would fidget through the class.

Now, in usual drama school style, students were asked to undertake group work ostensibly designed to facilitate group cohesion and honesty. In Ch1's case, their group was instructed to form a circle, then tell the group things about individuals in the group that they found annoying. Ch1 was told, repeatedly and in front of all their peers, that all these small behaviours were deeply irritating. They were criticized by students and staff for being fidgety and distracting. Having dyspraxia (coordination and motor skills issues) meant they had to work an awful lot harder than other students in many ways, yet they were told they were lazy and "made an example of" in front of the class. Making light of it, they would laugh at themselves, only to be wounded by the class joining in the laughter.

It seemed to us at the time there was no institution – from early years to university level – with even a basic level of knowledge about special needs. Special needs awareness was for special needs departments, which my children rarely encountered, and not for regular teachers who my children encountered on a daily basis. It was in this situation that my oldest child was forced to lead and advocate for themselves – and my leadership as a parent also had to take itself to yet another new educational setting.

The university knew all its legal rights regarding parents making contact and made our job of helping our child very difficult. Eventually, we were allowed to attend a meeting but for the next two years our oldest child was forced to lead and advocate for themselves, with varying success. For instance, the casual use of the racial slur "N" word was only confronted years later when Ch1 left and felt they were empowered enough to face the institution and call it out as wrong. Ch1 has found their "leader voice".

Leading for Ch4: Not all SEN are the same

And finally, a look at the early journey of Ch4 and what I had to do to lead in his care. To a certain extent, things should have been easier for Ch4, as he was adopted and therefore already on the school's radar. Unfortunately, he struggled from day one. Overwhelmed with complex, overlapping issues, it was almost impossible to work out how he was experiencing school and why things were going so very wrong. His physical age was equal to his actual age, but his emotional age was way behind. Feeling overwhelmed with 30 children in the class, he found it hard to do anything. He wasn't interested in reading, being read to, writing or even forming letters, guessing colours or animals, or painting – none of it interested him. He just wanted to feel safe and his whole day seemed to be focused on achieving this. He would climb into small spaces or try to escape the classroom; when he was prevented from doing so, it would lead to massive violent outbursts.

It became a liability having him in the classroom. Having watched all my children go through this same school, it was very interesting for us to watch the reaction to it. On the whole, I would say that this time there was a lot to praise in the leadership of the school as things began to melt down around Ch4. There were serious incidents, and the response to these incidents was right and fair. We entered into a whole new arena: this wasn't simply being unable to sit still, it was teachers with injuries, and absconding and setting the fire alarm off, leading to a whole-school evacuation. However, instead of simply blaming my child (which is how reactions to my older children had sometimes felt), the head of the school set up meetings with the Local Authority to gain more access to help. She pulled together all kinds of assistance and embraced new ideas. We truly had a collaborative approach.

Of course, there's no magic bullet, and school remained a huge challenge. The hardest part for Ch4 was that the school had no place to physically put him if he was unable to stay in the classroom, so for two years he and a series of TAs would take up residency in the school gym, where he would do his work and play.

The biggest issue for us, at this point, was other parents. The serious incidents meant Ch4 had the worst reputation you can imagine, and even though there were many good days, he could never come back from this image of being violent, out of control and a danger to all. He was six years old.

David and I dropped our child off to school and picked him up every day, so we were always present at the school classroom door at drop-off and pick-up times. Unbeknown to us, some other parents wanted to talk about the problem of our child. Even though our child was out of the classroom all day at this point, they had an issue with him being in the school at all. Apparently one parent decided to start a WhatsApp group for the parents in the class to join so they could talk about Ch4. Obviously, David and I were never invited to join. I was later told that his teacher (who was a relative of one of the parents) had recommended that the parents present a petition to have our son taken out of the school.

At first, I knew nothing of any of this. It wasn't until, in a meeting with the professionals involved in Ch4's care, the head talked about being presented with a petition that I became aware that any of this groundswell of hostility was happening. All the professionals seemed to know about it, though. I sat reeling in shock – not least because the people who had been in my home celebrating our family birthdays, people who I had thought of as friends, people who I had fought for in the school in the past because of their sexuality, had been the ones to present this petition on behalf of the class parents. It was devastating.

As the weeks went by, there were small moments of solace. I had parents in their ones and twos come to me saying they had refused to be a part of the petition, and a couple of parents asking my son round to play with their children. I cannot tell you how grateful I was for these parents. Even though they were small in number, their kindness and acceptance were like a healing balm.

It was at this time that I realized this was truly where you are judged as a parent for the behaviour of your children. It was as though the whole family was responsible for every one of Ch4's actions. I came to realize a strange truth: that until the moment of adoption, the outside world has compassion for the neglected and/or abused child, but the moment they come into their "forever family", that family is judged and held responsible for any adverse behaviours. Seemingly, all neglect and abuse are forgotten, and adoption is seen as a magic panacea that should – if you are a "good enough" parent – instantly fix all the hurt, all the challenging or anti-social behaviour, and all the consequences of the harm that has been done in the child's life. I later found solace in other adoptive families who talked about walking their child into school:

"Oh, you've experienced the walk of shame then!"

I didn't even realize it was a thing.

For Ch4, the label of being a danger of monster-like proportions has been very hard to shift.

So how could the leadership of this particular situation have been different? Our family is incredibly open about what we all face and how we are experiencing life, so we have reflected on this question among ourselves. Looking back, I believe it could have been an opportunity for the following:

- To share with and educate parents on what it's like for some adopted children. My child won't be the only adopted child they or their children face – maybe we could have used our experience to help make future adoptees' lives a little easier.
- To give an outline of the challenges our child was facing. Just like with my older children, the key to dealing with challenging behaviour is to understand where it is coming from. Our child was not a monster: he was on constant high alert, in flight-or-flight mode and terrified of his environment.

Perhaps if other parents had understood this, they would have had more compassion for Ch4.

- To give explicit permission for parents to talk to us about how they felt. We were always more than open to discussion, and at that time we were the "go to" parents in the playground to talk about SEND issues regarding their own children. Perhaps, though, the hostility that other parents were feeling caused them to be unwilling or unable to bring their feelings to us – we might have explicitly invited this, thus fostering more open communication.

- To work together to make life safe and kinder for both their children and my child, remembering – if current discourse around younger generations is anything to go by – that these are the same children who will be accused of being snowflakes and having no resilience in a few years' time.

I do feel this was a missed opportunity for the "village" to gather around the child. It also cemented in our child's mind that he was a reject and a monster, and someone to be feared. This is an image he still has to live with – even years later.

What can I sum up from all of these experiences? What have I learned from being dropped into the deep of leading the way for my children? The most important lesson for me is that leadership should happen *with* people and not *to* people. It takes time and patience, and ultimately requires the greatest tool in the toolbox: collaboration.

Learning objective: Parenting a child with non-dominant identities

To begin to understand the impact of parenting a child with one or more non-dominant identities in a society that is skewed towards dominant identities, and to build on this understanding to challenge your own assumptions about others. To consider how to deal with your own feelings about collaborating with very different people and viewpoints, and think about what collaborating might look like if all participants are on an equal footing.

3
Collaboration

We cannot begin to think about collaboration without first looking at the *status* and *equality* of those collaborating.

We are living in a world that places great value in status – a world more interested in net worth than self-worth. Too often, our job title carries more weight than our character. In almost every school meeting about my children, as we gather around the table, I have been super-aware of the ranking system in place. Everyone whose professional standing is relevant to the meeting seamlessly stakes out the room and works out their rank, taking their place with confidence. As parents we are just that – parents. Any status we may have in the world through our job is completely worthless in this environment unless it pertains to education. We are functional, we carry no expertise, we no longer even have a name, we are simply "Johnny's Mum" ... and more often than not, we are even addressed as such.

This is, of course, reductive and unhelpful. In any given situation, when we gather around a table to talk, we all bring assets. We all bring something of value, we all have something to offer. We also often bring our histories, our insecurities, and our fears. It is only through good leadership of the team that we can move forward together – in other words, how we are led will dictate how successful we are at achieving good collaboration.

Finding our humanity in these situations is *vital*. We do not just bring our job or title to a meeting, we should be encouraged to bring all of who we are into everything we do. Where we find humanity, we find humility and its wonderful partner, empathy.

Child-centred collaboration

Understanding one another's viewpoint is fundamental to finding a strategy that works for the child. The phrase "child-centred collaboration" is often used, yet all too often I've found that these meetings are not about what works for the child, but rather what works for the school. But to me this is backwards: if school cannot work for the child, then what is school here for?

I have attended many meetings where those around the table look something like Figure 3.

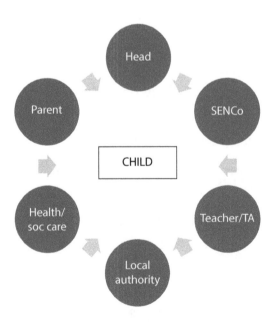

Figure 3 A child-centred meeting

This is the aim of the collaboration space. For the ultimate collaboration experience, every stakeholder (everyone who is impacted) should be present at the meeting. This means that for meetings about a child's education, the child or young person should always be present, even if just for part of the time. The more they are included in the development of plans, the more likely they are to embrace the changes and provisions that are made.

As for the other people in the room, the roles present can vary. You may have a virtual school head, a school governor, advocates, lawyers, union leaders, social workers, representatives from adoption services, autism specialists, speech and language specialists, and so on. It can be a big group, and it will vary massively depending on the child's circumstances. It always interests me, for example, that when I have meetings for my adopted child there are sometimes as many as 12 people in the room, while for my autistic children there might be perhaps three or four people – and I have never successfully been able to even hold a meeting about a child with ADHD. This is telling in itself. The adoption lobby is strong (and rightly so), and has been around for decades, so there is a lot more set up and in place for these children. We know that every child's needs are not the same – and this holds true for children with SEND. Not all SEND is the same, including when it comes to existing systems and provisions.

Barriers to child-centred collaboration

I have noticed certain challenges when trying to collaborate with professionals in this way. Although everyone usually wants to work towards the child-centred model described above, the reality is often different. There are plans, schemes, and desires that professionals may hold, which consciously or subconsciously can work against keeping the child and their needs in the centre of the thinking. Perhaps someone has come to the table with their own agenda. Maybe there's a lack of belief in the child or in the process. Often, there is simply not enough funding to do what everyone wants to do … and sometimes, sadly, the people in the room are all too exhausted, depleted, and overwhelmed to be effective. Then the meeting starts to look more like Figure 4:

Let's look at how this might play out. Here are some examples of the way various factors can de-centre a child from a meeting:

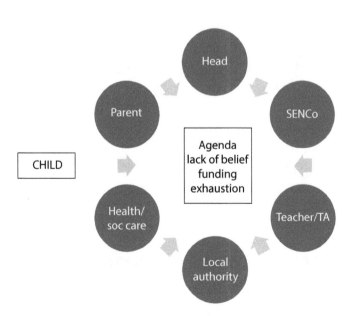

Figure 4 A child-centred meeting gone wrong

Agenda:

- A head of school wants the results of their school to be as high as possible. Focusing on the average grades may not motivate someone to help the child with learning differences, who may not get high grades no matter what resources are provided.
- The head may feel pressure from other parents, who feel their children are being held back by their peers with SEND.
- The head may feel that SEND children should be in SEND schools, and feel reluctant to help a child integrate.

Lack of belief:

- Some professionals simply cannot see the potential in the child.
- Some professionals doubt their own ability to make a difference.
- Conversely, some don't actually see the problem the child may be facing. I spent years being told that Ch2 was not autistic, despite the fact that we had a professional report showing a diagnosis of autism.

Funding:

- The Local Authority, the school, or CAMHS have spent their budget.
- The Local Authority or school have had their budget cut.
- What the child needs costs too much.
- The school thinks the Local Authority should cover the cost, while the Local Authority thinks the school should cover it.

- Professionals find it hard to tell the difference between equality and equity, and therefore deem the child undeserving of any budget allocation, even if the money is there.

Exhaustion:

- There may be a willingness to listen and act, but the professionals around the table are too worn down by the system, or so overloaded that they cannot engage in any meaningful way.
- The parents are so exhausted from fighting that they cannot believe that – or see how – they can represent their child

The mindset of collaboration

In the previous chapter, I described new-style leaders having the ability to say, "I don't know". This is important if we are to lead through change, and it becomes absolutely critical when we come to collaboration. True teamwork means being open to others, listening, and exhibiting that wonderful trait: curiosity.

Curiosity is a powerful thing. In a letter to his biographer, Albert Einstein wrote, "I have no special talents. I am only passionately curious [lit. passionate about new ideas]" (Einstein, 1952).

This is a beautiful concept of curiosity – passion for new ideas, new ways of doing things, new connections. Imagine if we all embraced curiosity as Einstein did! Unfortunately, being curious is all too often seen in a much more negative light. Here is an alternative view of curiosity from Vladimir Nabokov, as cited by author Azar Nafizi: "Curiosity is insubordination in its purest form" (Nafizi, 2003).

It is important to be able to accept that we are all learning. Even as I write this, I am aware of new discoveries, new preferences, changes to language, changes to policy, and so on. With every change comes new learning. Being curious about another's perspective is vital: we must listen through the words someone speaks and into the heart of what they are saying. Perhaps we are not all sophisticated communicators, but we can all work on our listening skills.

Boxed-in thinking

Having an open mindset is essential, and part of achieving that involves thinking outside the box. Most of us have boxed thinking in at least some areas of our lives, and this can limit us as we work together with others. Let's break down what feeds into boxed-in thinking.

Base: "only one way"

The base of the "box" is the foundation for everything in our mindset. Let's call this perceived truth or agreed traditions. When

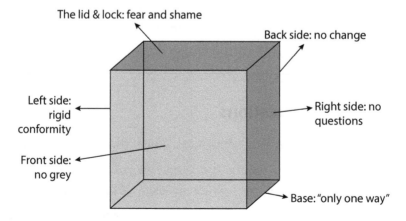

Figure 5 Boxed-in thinking

we are in the box, we all agree that we all share the same truth and have the same belief system and traditions – like the "one story" world I spoke about in Chapter 1. The base of the box says this: there is one way, and we all agree. You will generally recognize it when you encounter it – for example, with Ch3 in secondary school, I was constantly told that "school is an institution" by way of letting me know that any proposed changes would not be agreed to.

Back side: no change

This wall of the box says that there can be no change. Built on the foundation of "only one way", it follows that there can be no change: change is bad, change rocks the boat and undermines tradition, change is threatening and unnecessary. This is the way we have always done things, so it is the way we will continue. The institution must be served and upheld.

Left side: rigid conformity

This wall of the box builds on the base and leans on the back side. If there is only one way, and change is bad, then rigid conformity must follow. Anything other than rigid conformity is mocked, undermined and not to be trusted – because it is dangerous. We must all look, think, and be the same, because individuality of thought is seen as rebellion.

Right side: no questions

This wall mirrors the one opposite. While the left side says rigid conformity is necessary, the opposite wall reinforces the message by making sure questions are seen as impertinent and disrespectful. There can be no challenge. Questions undermine authority, and curiosity is seen as flagrant disregard for the proper way of doing things.

Front side: no grey

With all these walls in place, there can be no shades of difference in opinion. Black and white thinking, with its absolute certainty, is celebrated. Grey is seen as "shady".

The lid and lock: fear and shame

And how are people kept in their place inside the box? By fear. There is nothing like fear to silence people. Fear leaves us alienated and alone. And to really keep us trapped in boxed-in thinking, if fear is the lid then its partner shame is the lock. If you actually manage to get out of the box, it is the shaming that will have you rushing to jump back in.

See the problem? We all carry these boxes around with us about one thing or another – the key to teamwork is to deconstruct the box around that area of thinking. In other words, if we are to collaborate well, then we must first work on our mindset. There is joy and freedom to be found in breaking out of this box: collaboration is all about creativity, which is like play when done well and can be a wonderful thing when all parties are committed.

The ten assumptions of collaboration

One of the greatest challenges to collaboration is assumption. Unhelpful assumptions can be made by anyone. Parents and carers make assumptions, and so do professionals.

1. Parents have one child

There is often an assumption that parents have only one child, so all children are dealt with singularly. The reality, though, is that it is not unusual in families to have more than one person with SEN. Each child's life impacts the next child's life, and SEND parents are often jumping from one meeting to another, including experiencing diary clashes. Often there is a huge overlap in the services being delivered to parents, and there's a lot of repetition and redundancy. For instance, two of my children attend schools 30 and 40 minutes' drive away and the Local Authority provide transport with a chaperone. It's a big cost to the Local Authority. My children could travel in the same car, as both schools are on the same route, but this cannot be done because the systems are set up for one school/one car, so they travel separately.

2. Professionals have no outside life

It can be easy to assume, as a parent or carer, that professionals are literally just their job. But these people have lives, stresses, and joys, the same as everyone else. Across every service I have encountered, I have seen professionals who have come into the service with the aim of making a difference, only to find that a little while later they are ground down and have to take time off work for mental health reasons. I have known social worker teams where five members are down to two, and the service employs one temporary member of staff to cover them. Inevitably, within a few months, the two who are having to carry the full load end up off sick. The pressure on our professional services is extreme. As parents, we must remember that we are not the only ones facing pressure.

3. Parents are only parents

As a society, we really need to level up our view of parents. It is important to remember that parents – just like professionals – have many other facets to their personhood besides being parents, which can be potentially helpful to a child-centred collaboration, and can also be limiting factors that need to be taken into account. Here's how this doesn't work at the moment: as a person who has Crohn's Disease, I have often had to choose between a hospital appointment for myself and a CAMHS appointment for my child that I have been waiting for months for. I have had to face school demands regarding one child while sitting on suicide watch in hospital with another child. Unfortunately, my children do not schedule their meltdowns or breakdowns!

4. Parents don't get it and are not expert

Some of the most "expert" people I have encountered are actually the parents of the child. Parents often understand their children on a very deep level; they have known the child the longest and spent more time with the child than anyone else. I have also encountered parents who have been fighting for so long that they understand law and human rights, and have incredible medical knowledge. Plus, some parents will actually be professionals themselves – remember, we are all more than one thing. It can be easy to dismiss a parent who has never studied for a medical or educational degree, but it's important not to discount the expertise of lived experience.

5. Professionals can solve everything

Managing the expectations of parents can sometimes be a challenge, especially if the parents are struggling with their child's diagnosis. It is important to let parents know what is possible and why, and what may not be possible and why.

6. Parents don't want to engage

I hear teacher friends say this a lot. I have never met a parent who didn't want to engage with school over their child's needs, but I know they must exist – and I imagine that working with those parents is a different piece of work that needs to be undertaken. This is where whole family support really comes in. However, it is important not to assume that parents don't care or don't want to be involved. As I said, I have never met a parent who didn't.

7. Parents are *too* engaged

On the other hand, we have the notion that parents who do get involved are a pain, an obstacle, something to be "handled" rather than a fellow collaborator. An engaged parent is a gift. "Warrior" parents like me are forged in the furnace of affliction. Being ignored and overlooked while watching your child fall to pieces will do that to you – so don't waste the passion, the expertise, the strength and stamina that a truly engaged parent will bring. Often, no one wants to find a successful collaboration more than a child's parent, so please don't write them off as an annoyance.

8. All families have white, English, neurotypical thinking

Professionals need a basic understanding of people of different cultures, faiths, sexualities, genders, disabilities, neuro-divergences, and so on. Even within the group of "white, English, neurotypical" there is a lot of variation! People communicate in different ways and have different worldviews. There is also sometimes the assumption that people have the money to pay for computers, phones, and separate rooms in their homes to have a quiet place to speak. I can think of one clear example that we encountered of this bias, in one friend of ours who during the COVID-19 pandemic, with seven children and one device, was meant to facilitate her children's online education.

9. Everyone has lots of time on their hands

We all need to appreciate the time restraints that people have. Teachers already work long hours; many professionals have huge caseloads; and most parents will also be trying to hold down a job as well as make all the school-hours meetings. Grace and understanding are a must.

10. The problem is money

It would be harmful and wrong to simply think that throwing enough money at a situation is always the answer – and it's definitely counter to true collaboration. I have encountered meetings where the issue of funding has been discussed, of course, but overwhelmingly, the issue at hand is almost always more about mindset than money.

The ten markers of good collaboration
1. All stakeholders are present

As I said before, everyone impacted by a meeting's outcome should be present at the meeting, and everything should be done to make that happen. I tire of hearing how a group of neurotypical people is debating how an autistic person is experiencing the world, or how exclusively white people are telling Black people what it's like to be Black. The more we listen, the more we can become good allies. There is something very special about meetings where you know everyone who has any power to change things sits alongside those who need to see that change. A few years ago, I went to make a speech to a Local Authority of about 200 leaders. The speech before mine was a leader speaking about the need to reach into the Bangladeshi Community. Apparently, they had 2,000 Bangladeshi people in their borough. When it was my turn to speak, I asked how many of the leaders in the room were Bangladeshi. The answer, as I knew it would be, was none. I then asked, "So out of 2,000 people, are you telling me there isn't one person with leadership potential?" It's a simple concept, but one that is routinely ignored: nothing about us without us.

2. All are of equal status

Flatten the hierarchy and give value to all.

3. Everyone understands the language, which is kind

If you are a professional, remember you have gradually changed the way you speak about your work and about children. There are words and phrases you use that parents and those with SEND may not understand. Rather than saying, "We need a robust pathway", try "We need to find a plan that works." Using common language means we all get a chance to take part. Professionals need to be mindful of the power of their words and the impact they can have. Parents are not professionals; they are deeply emotionally connected to the situation.

I had a meeting once where two girls had bullied Ch2, sending multiple messages on Snapchat telling my child to kill themselves. This was at a time when my child was constantly suicidal and in and out of hospital. My husband and I attended a meeting to talk things through and we spoke about our child feeling isolated and friendless. In response, the head told us that this was to be expected; he said that when autistic teenagers get to this age they lose friends and end up alone. We felt absolutely devastated by his words. They weren't even true; his opinion has no basis in fact and we knew that, but they were words intended to hurt, and hurt they did. Those years were so very hard in every way. Facing such opposition when we were also facing the most difficult situation we had ever faced as parents was brutal – just what we didn't need when we didn't know whether our child would live to see 16 years of age.

4. Everyone has a chance to speak

Professionals are used to representing their views, but parents and those with SEND are often not, especially at the outset of the journey. Great collaboration happens when we allow people to speak in the language that works best for them. Pictures, paintings, poems, and video can all be used. Sometimes a picture can literally paint a thousand words – but there has to be space and the technology for that communication to happen.

5. Everyone is heard

It's one thing to take in sounds, but quite another to really *hear* someone. Hearing happens with our ears, minds, and hearts; good hearing is laced with an empathy that translates what the speaker is trying to communicate. There is no shame in checking to see whether what you are "hearing" is correct. Checking allows the speaker to elaborate and sometimes even work out what it is they are trying to say.

When Ch2 was 15 years old, we had to update their old statement into an EHCP. It was the most painful process, with blocks to change at every move and no will to make things work. In fact, the person in school who was responsible for creating the EHCP had one general meeting with me about Ch2 and how things were going, and I was later told the creation of the EHCP had occurred that day. It was presented as a fait accompli. It meant I was terribly nervous about getting mine and Ch2's voice heard. I had to fill out a form to record Ch2's opinion of things – something which can be very difficult for anyone, let alone a young person who struggles with communication.

I decided I would interview them on camera at home. I had never edited footage, never used iMovie, and I am not particularly technically aware. But I dived in anyway: I edited the film, added photographs of their art, music they loved, and footage of them dancing. They looked straight into the camera and shared what would work for them and all the things they wished that teachers would know and understand about them. I was so pleased with what we had managed to create – something that clearly communicated and felt positive.

As I entered the meeting, though, I could feel the atmosphere. It was hostile. They had gathered extra staff to be present so that I was completely outnumbered and alone. I asked if I could play the filmed piece before we began, and thankfully they agreed. It was an utterly compelling piece of evidence, and the mood of the room shifted completely. In this video, the voice of the young person at the centre of things was heard and it set the tone for the whole meeting. It was only at this point, some four years into our SEN journey with Ch2, that I felt we were being truly heard for the first time. They could argue with me as a parent, they could undermine me, criticize me, take away my right to speak to teachers – but finally, *finally*, I had shown that they could not silence my child. It was a real victory. From that day, things slowly began to change.

There is also nothing wrong with repeating what is being said in a meeting, to make sure everyone understands and is on the same page. I recently had a wonderful meeting at Ch4's school. It is a school that is committed to working alongside parents, and has incredible humanity and compassion towards the child. A few times in the meeting I said, "What I'm hearing is …" This phrase, and the action of repeating back in my own words, really helped the meeting to move forward. People had a chance to correct what they had said if I had heard something they did not mean, and the chance to affirm my understanding if it was correct. In fact, this was the meeting at which I found out my son's placement was no longer working, and that he would have to leave the school. But you'll note I described it as wonderful!

The point is this: even painful conversations can happen and happen well if the relationships are strong. When people are heard, it makes for good collaboration and it makes everything a whole lot easier – even the hard stuff.

6. We can all sit with discomfort

Learning to sit with discomfort is one of the biggest assets we can possess. When we can tolerate what is being said to us, no matter how uncomfortable it may be, we can work out what to do next in a measured way. If we cannot tolerate discomfort in ourselves, we will always hand the power to the next person. If we cannot tolerate discomfort in others, then we'll always try to placate and ameliorate, and this can lead to bad decisions being made. Robust conversations are often a necessity. We have to be able to look at where things are going wrong, even if we are the ones responsible for the situation. Good collaboration often has some very awkward moments – and that's okay.

In an early meeting I had for Ch4 in primary school, when those involved were just getting to know us, I had an interaction that brought some discomfort into to the room. It was at a point when the school needed to do more. A member of the CAMHS team came to the meeting and suggested family therapy in the shape of parent work for my husband and me. Now, I am always up for some learning, but I knew that this comment at this time was intended to deflect away from the need for the school to take on more responsibility – in other words, it was an attempt to "pass the buck". By this time, I knew how to advocate for myself and my child quite well, so I made it clear that we wouldn't be doing parent work. I was then taken to one side by the therapist and told that I would get no help from anyone if I didn't "play the game" – an attitude that did him no credit at all. He hated finding himself in the midst of a robust conversation with me disagreeing with him, and his inability to bear the discomfort led to very strange behaviours for a professional.

7. New ideas are welcome

This is again about all of us being open to change. If we are thinking outside the box, the potential for creativity is limitless. I have lost count of the number of meetings I have been in where ideas have been shut down immediately simply because the idea has never been done before.

8. Good ideas can come from anywhere

Everyone is creative; anyone can have a good idea. When status is flattened, it allows for those good ideas to come forth. Often people who are a little more distanced from the situation can come up with great ideas, sometimes because they do not have an awareness of the blocks to change that exist, or sometimes because they are using pre-existing skills from another area of their lives. Some of the best ideas I have heard about have come from teaching assistants. Those who work face to face, closely with the children, have a good idea of what works and what doesn't, yet it is rare to find a TA in a professionals' collaboration meeting.

9. Everyone understands what they have to do moving forward

Many meetings I attend are not minuted, and this means good ideas can be lost or the same things end up being discussed again at the next meeting. There should be a sense of forward motion with ideas. If everyone understands their responsibilities to the situation, it means the workload can be shared fairly and everyone gets to play their part. It is rarely the job of one person to solve all the issues, yet this is often what happens. Sometimes this is the expectation from the rest of the collaborators, and sometimes it lies with a person who feels only they can properly solve the issues. The best work is achieved when people work together in teams.

10. Ideas are followed up, failure is allowed, and we work until it works

Parents will tell you that sometimes they manage to get a brilliant EHCP, only to find the school aren't applying the provision laid out in the plan. It is important that everyone follows the plan, and that the successes and failures of the plan are regularly reviewed and adjusted. We all know what can happen to the best-laid plans – reviews are important.

The area of provision for our SEND cohort is often hit and miss. The cohort is made up of people, not diagnoses, and people are individuals. We can think we've come up with the perfect plan on paper only to find that the person doesn't want to or cannot engage with it at all. It is then that we have to go back to the drawing board. Failing forward means we learn from the experience, and we adapt things until we find something that works. This takes time and effort, and the will to get it right. Matthew Syed has a great book about this, called *Black Box Thinking: The Surprising Truth About Success (and Why Some People Never Learn from Their Mistakes)* (Syed, 2015).

Earlier this year, I hosted an awards ceremony for a pharmaceutical company. I was stunned and delighted to see that a category had appeared that I have never seen in any awards ceremony before: the "Best Failed Project" category. There were a number of teams competing for the prize. The point of the award was to see who had learned the most from the failure of a project – what an amazing approach to collaboration and innovation! The road to success is often paved with failure. The question to ask is: What can I take from this experience to use as a building block for future success?

Learning objective: Holistic education plan

To consider how to make a plan for a young person's education that is holistic and meets their needs on an ongoing basis, even as that child's needs change and evolve, by making sure you take the time to get to know the young person and their needs and strengths properly.

4
Strategy

Who is the plan for?

Now let's look at strategy. We'll consider how to find the best strategies, and how those strategies are embedded in lives and schools. But first, when making a plan, it is always important to remember who the plan is *for*, so you can make sure the plan works for them.

Form and flow

There has been a lot of talk in leadership circles over the decades about a concept called "form and flow", where form is a very structured plan that all adhere to, and flow is seeing what's happening around you and responding. This narrative has come from two key contributors, Porter and Mintzberg.

Porter is known for competitive strategy; the idea here is to look at how everybody else is doing things, then use that knowledge to make your company better than what is already out there (Porter, 1979). The challenge to this methodology was that it could only ever look in a backward direction, and didn't allow for the emerging globalization and advanced technology breakthroughs that would have business moving at a much quicker rate. The structure was good and necessary, but with a rear-view outlook, the structure didn't have the agility needed to move forward quickly and adapt to constant change.

On the other hand, Mintzberg's "emergent strategy" sums up the concept of a flow strategy so well: it describes the process of recognizing and formalizing a business strategy that has not necessarily been planned, but has emerged more organically (Mintzberg, 1987). Interestingly, Mintzberg also argues that a successful strategy is never purely planned/proactive nor purely emergent/reactive – he suggests that strategy is always a combination of both.

The point is that we can come with the most fabulous strategies and structures in the world, but if we are not flexible and do not have the agility to observe and go with the flow, we will never meet the needs of our SEND children. Plans are great. Plans set the tone – I am never going to suggest that we don't have a plan. Having a good framework is essential … but frankly, plans are not worth the paper they are written on if they *do not work for the child*. Every strategy should be accompanied by the flexible outlook that considers:

- every child is different;
- every child is evolving;
- the world is continually evolving too; and
- children belong in families – there is always a bigger picture than just the child.

It's a daily update. Of course, we must create the framework from what we already know, but we can only meet the needs of our children if we are able to notice the emerging differences and flow with the changes. This is where the collaboration rubber hits the road. If we have created something that is largely workable, then add to it agility and good communication between all parties concerned and quick adjustments can be made. If every change demands a meeting and signing off by all parties, the child will fade before change ever arrives.

Every child is different

I cannot stress this enough. What autism looks like in different people can be incredibly contrasting. Ch2 wants to get everything right and obey every rule, while Ch3 doesn't care about rules and needs convincing of even the most basic of demands. Ch2 as incredible attention to detail in every aspect of life, whereas Ch3 overlooks details and their life is instead led by feelings and having their needs met.

In fact, autism does not even always look the same in the *same* person on a day-to-day basis, let alone between different people. On one day, Ch2 may be fully confident and able to engage with everyone in any situation. The next day, they may not be able to make eye contact or speak, and the thought of being sociable is terrifying. It is clear that there needs to be a flexible plan that wraps around the child. The plan serves the child; the child doesn't serve the plan.

Every child is evolving

Individual change is important to recognize on a number of levels; ideally, you will be able to think in advance about how children may respond to change.

Developmental change

There are developmental stages in a child's life, both physically and mentally. As our bodies and brains develop, some things become easier and some things can become harder. Suddenly a child may be able to tolerate something they would have run away from a year before. Or equally, hormones arrive and suddenly we appear to face a whole new child. The strategies we have around our children should reflect these changes.

Intersections

Children, like all people, have intersectional identities. Factors such as their race, sexuality, and gender can interact in different ways, and new things may crop up in the development of their identity at any time. What children need more than anything is the space to explore these questions and feelings that they may have; this is true for all children, but a child who has SEND may experience things differently from their peers. For instance, one study has found that transgender and gender-diverse people (such as those who identify as non-binary, like some of my children) are three to six times as likely to be autistic as cisgender people (Warrier et al., 2020), so it is worth bearing this in mind as we seek to understand our autistic cohort. Where a child's greatest challenge may in the past have been anxiety, it may now be gender dysphoria (the condition of feeling one's emotional and psychological identity to be at variance with one's birth sex), or for some it may be difficult to separate the two.

Identity

As our children grow, they develop new ideas about themselves. They become excavators of personality, style, and beliefs, speeding along in the journey of self-discovery. Young people find things they love and hate about themselves. Once puberty hits, it is a time of deep reflection. We know our children can be harsh critics of their parents, but harsher than anything for them is the voice of the inner critic. It is at this stage of maturing that young people may develop unhelpful or problematic behaviours, so the plans and strategies for children may change.

The world is continually evolving

This is self-evident – we know that the world is always changing and moving on. There may be global disruptions, as we have seen with COVID-19. The pandemic of 2020–2022 (ongoing at the time of writing) has challenged all school pupils and teachers alike. Online learning, independent learning, catching up, isolation, anxiety, and fear of death – all these things impact everyone in school, of course, but perhaps even more deeply for our SEND cohort. How does the plan look when schooling is disrupted? How does the plan respond now schooling is being resumed?

There are also more known changes in the world, such as climate change and technological advancements. These things can have an impact on how a school does things in both a positive and negative way. How might these ongoing issues affect the plan?

Then there are the smaller scale, personal life experiences and events that maybe don't change the whole world, but do change a child's world. Children come from families or home set-ups. The death of a close relative, seeing your birth parents for the first time, having a parent in hospital, having a sibling in hospital, being permanently excluded from school – these are all experiences our family has faced, and I can see how they have shaped our children's lives and worldviews, and how their needs have changed accordingly.

Who are you?

So, what's the first step to developing a strategy that is both planned and emergent, both proactive and reactive, and that will work with and for a child through all these changes? First, we must be on a continual journey of getting to know the person for whom that plan is made. In the background of everything, I am always attempting to find out who my children are. When I find clues to their evolving personalities and identities, I can encourage this.

It might sound daunting, but it's really just an extension of how many of us naturally relate to children. Most people have at some point asked a child of their acquaintance, "What do you want to be when you grow up?" Perhaps you remember being asked this question yourself. Of course, children have all kinds of magical ideas, and usually name one of about five jobs they can think of – from the sublime to the ridiculous. This question is a common one and can help adults understand the children in their lives, as the answer to the question changes through time. But we can go a step further: my preferred question to ask my children is this:

"Who are you, and who and what are you here for?"

When a person finds their purpose, it goes way beyond a job title. When purpose flows from identity, the person has a greater chance of achieving life satisfaction and, where there are also good relationships, wholeness too. Purpose is linked to who and what we care about. It is linked to making a difference to our world, however small or large – and from a surprisingly young age, children can engage with the question at a level that works for them.

Child 1

Ch1 is wise, funny, sensitive, creative, artistic, an insightful listener, and good at planning and executing ideas. They love people, the arts, and travel. Their purpose, I'm sure, will be found in something that brings some or all of these areas together.

Every child is different

One of the areas we have had to navigate with Ch1 is that there could well be overlapping traits. Autism, ADHD, trauma, anxiety disorders, and probably many other neurodevelopmental conditions have overlapping areas. At the age of 27, Ch1 is now considering getting assessed for autism as well as having ADHD. Let me repeat this: even though I have two children with clear autistic diagnoses, both of whom are different from each other, it has taken Ch1 until adulthood before they and we considered that they might also be autistic. The point is that even within families, we can easily overlook a person's difference because it doesn't look like what we are used to. Every child is different; it's so easy to forget.

Every child is evolving

Two years ago, when Ch1 came out to me as non-binary, it was a very subtle approach. So subtle, in fact, that I missed it. We were in the kitchen. I was cooking, they were sitting at the kitchen table. I sensed no change in the atmosphere; I was completely unaware that my child was trying to communicate with me. Sometimes we can be in the room geographically but not present in the moment – and the more exhausted we are, the more this can happen. It's a survival tactic. This must have been one such time. Ch1 was doodling in a notebook when suddenly they turned the book towards me. I looked down. It was a blank page except for one sentence, which read,

"I am non-binary."

I had no idea of the implications of this statement, and because of this it didn't feel like a big deal, so I simply answered,

"That's lovely, darling."

A year later their younger sibling, Ch2, came out as non-binary too, and I went into discovery mode, hoping I could become an ally and a great supporter. Looking back, I feel that I really failed my older child; to a certain extent, I had forgotten they had even come out, and it took another child coming out to remind me and prompt me to get to know what this aspect of my children's identities meant. Again, it's so easy to forget – we think we know our children, but every child is constantly evolving and we must *keep* getting to know them as this happens.

The world is continually evolving

Having a suicidal sibling can be nullifying, and can lead to overwhelming feelings of being overlooked. It can lead to feeling that even though your needs are great, their needs are greater, and no one is noticing yours. All eyes are on the emergency. The time and energy spent on keeping Ch2 alive and in school meant that Ch1 had less attention. Ch1 was by no means ignored, but Ch2 had more than normal amounts of intense attention, which left Ch1 feeling that they were not allowed to have problems. In their mind, they believed we as parents may not be able to cope with anything more. They could see how much Ch2 needed us, and how much we gave – and they didn't want to be a burden.

There's lot to unpick here. First, what happens when we fail our children? The stakes seem very high and recovery feels unsurmountable, but thankfully the human heart is often more resilient than we realize. Asking for our child's forgiveness is an important experience on the parenting journey – for us, it was an essential part of the plan for Ch1.

***

Responding to gender identity

I want to take a moment here to reflect on one specific way that a child's plan might need to adapt: that of their gender identity. What I have learned from my non-binary children coming out to me is that I have much to learn; and I am beyond willing to do so. It's not an area I had really ever thought about before it was brought to me, but I have learned that it's very important for us to understand. Ch1's pronouns are they and them. This is something I really struggled to get on top of to begin with, but my children helped me to understand a few things:

- My annoyance at myself when I misgender my children only makes them feel bad. They have had to go through enough to get to this point, so I need to "get out of the way" and not make it about me. If I misgender them, I apologize, correct myself and move on, or simply correct myself and move on. Never over-apologize.

- I have noticed a trend where people refer to my children as they/them – the correct pronouns – when they are in the room, but if they aren't present, then the speaker reverts back to using she/her – which is not correct. This is *really* disrespectful, because it somehow implies that the speaker is "humouring" my children rather than respecting their identity. Switching up like this also makes the whole process of learning to use the correct pronouns drag out even longer. Let's be clear: a non-binary person isn't non-binary only when they are with you; they are non-binary all of the time. How we speak about people when they are not there is very telling of how we value them – and that includes the pronouns we use.

- Being non-binary is not something that people choose in order to be "trendy" or "woke". There is nothing advantageous about it when you are bullied, trolled, and constantly misgendered. The non-binary people I have met all have extraordinary stories of struggle; many of them have had to struggle with gender dysphoria, including terrible feelings about themselves and their body. Who would choose this for themselves?

- Non-binary people do not owe it to us to have to explain their existence every day. They are not educators on the subject, and they have enough to deal with without becoming some kind of unwitting representative for all non-binary and trans people. The responsibility for learning lies on us. As my kids always say, "Google is free." If we are interested in learning, then our natural curiosity can be met online, where there is plenty to see and read.

- I have never heard as many debates over difference as I have about gender. Everyone seems to have an opinion on the matter, even if they have never actually met a non-binary person. People complaining about having to use different pronouns, saying it doesn't work grammatically or offends their sense of good grammar. Honestly! It's a small change for us, but it makes a big difference to the non-binary person. Besides – the singular "they" has been around in English for a long, long time, and is in no way grammatically incorrect. My editor confirmed it!

- Non-binary people do not have to dress in an androgenous style to help us understand them or to be valid. Try not to make assumptions about people based on whether you think they dress "feminine" or "masculine" enough.

- Sometimes a non-binary person may change their name, as three of my children have. When a trans or non-binary person chooses a new name, the name they were given at birth is then known as their "dead name". Calling someone by their dead name can really cause hurt; we may have feelings about the name that we first knew someone with, whether that's our child or a young person we work with, but I guarantee you our feelings about their name are not as strong or as important as *their* feelings about their name. What we call each other matters a great deal, so it is important to be respectful.

- Sexuality and gender are not the same thing. Non-binary people are included in the transgender group, the "T" of LGBTIQ+. Just because someone is non-binary, it's important we don't make assumptions about their sexual orientation.

- Being non-binary is not a "third gender"; the concept of non-binary generally implies a spectrum as opposed to – well, a binary! There are many shades to gender; non-binary people are not trying to add a third category to a two-category system, but rather are stepping outside of the binary altogether.

- This is nothing new. Non-binary people have existed for thousands of years in many ancient cultures and there is much written about this – it's not a new fad, or a young people's trend that they will get over; it's an extremely normal part of the rainbow of humanity.

If you want to learn more about non-binary identity, one resource I found particularly helpful is by the Oasis Charitable Trust. It's available for schools to use, and I found it great as a parent. You can find it by searching on the Oasis Charitable Trust website, here: www.oasisuk.org.

***

Child 2

Ch2 is gentle, magical, strong, determined, creative, artistic, complex, curious, a great friend, loyal, and truthful. Their purpose will be found in this.

Every child is different

Earlier in the book, we've looked a little at the different present-ations of autism that can be seen in different individuals. Here, I'd like to focus on a really common misconception: empathy. The common stereotype is that autistic people lack empathy entirely, and can never understand other people's feelings – that they in fact lack emotions altogether. Of course, the truth is a lot more complex than this. It's certainly untrue that all autistic people lack emotion and empathy – I know that from experience – but what does the research say?

Professor Simon Baron-Cohen has done a lot of work around the "theory of mind" (the mind's ability to think about the mind) and autism. A 1994 study led by Baron-Cohen found that young autistic children struggle to recognize mental state words such as "think", "know", "dream", "pretend", "hope", "wish", and "imagine" from a long list of different words. This (along with other studies) suggested to the researchers that autistic people have difficulties with the theory of mind (thinking about thinking and feeling and lying); in the 1994 study, the researchers went on to try to isolate where in the physical brain these connections might be made (Baron-Cohen et al., 1994). In an article from 2000, Baron-Cohen writes that: "Difficulty in understanding other minds is a core cognitive feature of autism spectrum conditions" (Baron-Cohen, 2000). This probably led to the current stereotype that autistic people don't understand feelings.

But this is an over-simplification. Empathy isn't just about understanding the way the brain works – it's also about emotional connection. For neurotypical people, a good proxy for measuring emotional connection is eye contact – the eyes are talked about as the windows of the soul. Again, the common stereotype of autistic people is that they will never look you in the eye – something that is seen as shifty, untrustworthy, and lacking in emotional connection. In the 1990s, there was a lot of academic focus on what the eyes did and how autistic people interpret another's gaze (Baron-Cohen and Cross, 1992; Baron-Cohen et al., 1995) – again, we have ended up with another stereotype that leads to all autistic people being seen as incapable of feelings and empathy.

But eye contact is only a proxy for how we understand connection – it isn't connection itself – and eye contact can fit in very differently with people who make connections in different ways. For example, eye contact may be distracting for me if I am reading you with my "gut". Or perhaps eye contact feels intensely intimate for me, and I am in fact trying to be polite by refusing to invade your personal space in that way. Both my autistic children make a lot of eye contact, as it happens, and although we haven't done a huge amount of talking about their individual theories of mind, I can definitely tell you that neither of them is emotionless or lacks empathy.

There has been a lot of work about the mind and the brain, but where there appears to be very little study is the "felt space" – our sense of others. This is sometimes referred to as being able to read situations with our "knower" or "gut instinct" – it might even be called our "sixth sense" – and this is where I see my autistic children flourish. As a performer and coach, gut instinct has been a finely honed tool for me for years, and has been invaluable in every area of my work. It helps me feel why connection is happening, or not happening, between a performer and an audience. It is something many of us use – and I think it's an important distinction to make.

Let's explore what that might look like. While I know that sometimes Ch2 struggles to understand why a friendship is going wrong – perhaps demonstrating this difficulty with theory of mind that Baron-Cohen identifies – Ch2 is also unbelievably perceptive, often feeling an issue long before anyone is showing any real signs of there being anything wrong. So, while they may not know why someone is feeling or thinking something, they will sense the feeling long before a neurotypical person might. From a young age, they have been able to feel other people's sadness, fear, anger, and kindness. This can happen before the person has spoken, or even if the person is presenting a very different emotion from the one they are actually feeling. Because of this finely tuned, sensitive "gut instinct", Ch2 is the go-to person to confide in among their friendship groups. They care, they want to help, they have incredible compassion – that doesn't sound like a lack of empathy or emotion to me.

This brings me full circle back to the point that every child is different, including every autistic child. Some may struggle with empathy, while others may have incredibly attuned empathy but struggle to understand it. Some may prefer not to make lots of eye contact, while others may be perfectly comfortable looking you in the eye. Let's not make a plan that is based on assumptions about how "autistic people are" – let's make a plan that is based on knowing the child in question.

Every child is evolving

I am always amazed at the sudden progress young people can make. Sometimes a life experience unlocks a whole new world for a person – activities or situations that may be impossible at one point are suddenly possible.

Ruth Fidler is a specialist in pathological demand avoidance (PDA) and has done some incredible work looking at the relationship between toleration and demand (Duncan et al., 2011). To build on this, I think it's important to include anxiety: in my experience, anxiety has a very strong relationship with the other areas of toleration and demand.

When Ch2's anxiety is high, their toleration levels decrease, making it difficult to place demands on them at these times. Discerning what is happening with their anxiety is therefore essential. Anxiety is not always attached to a particular situation, but might be rising at a background level. For a person with anxiety, it is sitting there at all times and will often simply attach itself to whatever is on their mind. It is this background anxiety that I try to concentrate on. What is it about their broader view of their life that they are struggling with? Underlying fears about

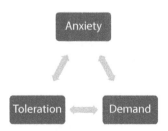

Figure 6 The anxiety cycle

themselves, relationships or work – all of these things can create high anxiety levels.

Here's an example of how the three factors can play out. Ch2 was set to make a new start in a new school. It was the beginning of Year 7, and the children were treated very gently as they transitioned from their primary settings into a much bigger, young adult world. Homework was set, but not too much of it. At this early stage, Ch2 managed to complete the homework – but was desperate to please, so would spend hours working on it to clearly unsustainable levels. By Term 2, everyone was expected to have settled into the school and so they introduced detentions. Any piece of homework not handed in on time would result in a detention for the student. Then they upped the stakes. Any class where a majority of students did not complete their homework on time would receive a whole-class detention. Suddenly, Ch2 could not avoid getting detention – even if they worked every spare hour on their own homework, they had no control over the others in their class. They developed high levels of fear of getting things wrong, or being punished for things they hadn't done. There were detentions for wrong school uniform, for being in the wrong place, for walking down a wrong corridor, for arriving late. Every single error was punishable. The environment this created for Ch2 was one of war-like proportions: "How do I make sure I do everything right? What happens if I do something wrong and I don't even know I'm doing something wrong? The teacher looks cross, the teacher doesn't like me, the teacher is going to humiliate me in front of the class, the teacher is going to make me stay behind." School became absolutely intolerable.

A few weeks into Term 2, Ch2 began to show signs of depression and high levels of anxiety.

Added to this was the growing issue of friendships. In the first term, there were lots of new people who were all a little scared and finding groups to hang out with in order to feel safe and befriended. In Term 2, the pairing off began and "best friendships" were formed. Like the unchosen child in the school sports team, Ch2 found themselves without a "best friend". By Term 3, the bullying had started (a sadly common experience for children with SEND). With a desperate need to fit in and be liked, they couldn't tell if they were saying the right thing. By Year 8, Ch2 was sinking deeper, and by Year 9, at age thirteen, they no longer wanted to live.

They had gone from anxiously acceding to demands – working for more hours than necessary on their homework in Term 1 of Year 7 – to being unable to tolerate even the smallest of demands, including even attending school at all. They were labelled a "school-refuser". I hate this term: it places the onus of responsibility on the child. In truth, it was the school that was doing the "refusing". It was not prepared to make the reasonable adjustments that would make school life tolerable for Ch2 – to allow them to manage their anxiety levels, thereby increasing their tolerance and ability to meet demands.

Thus began the period of Ch2's life I have already described: hospital visits, suicide watch, desperately trying to access help and support. Eventually, their health began to improve, and the turning point for this was no more and no less than a demand-free life. The only demand we made on Ch2 was to stay alive; anything else was forgotten. Most of the time they could tolerate nothing more than being in their bedroom, a few interactions with family, and the lowest levels of self-care. But with time and no demands, their tolerance gradually increased. By the age of 16, they were managing to get into school – albeit only for a couple of hours a day, and not every day. Then came the most significant change for Ch2: into this scene of extremely low tolerance and low demands – after many, many battles, calls, tears, struggles, and pleas – they were granted the support they needed from the school. Having a TA coming to the home proved to be just what Ch2 needed. Suddenly, they were able to get into school more often – because they knew they had this arrangement as a fallback, which lowered their anxiety levels straight away. In turn, this meant their toleration increased so demands could also increase. We had the breakthrough we had been waiting for. Our child was evolving and changing, and the strategy they needed evolved with them.

The world is continually evolving

From a bedroom-sized world, to visits from the TA, to making it into school more regularly – all these experiences were the small wins that were gigantic in our lives. And then we had the world-changing experience of Ch2 getting a job at the age of 16: the first Black autistic actor and the first person assigned female at birth to play an autistic role in a UK TV drama.

As they began to emerge from their bedroom life, it was important that we were still "checking in" on how they were doing with anxiety and making any adjustments necessary. Their employer made lots of adjustments to help them manage their anxiety, and within a few months, Ch2 found themselves able to travel on trains, stay away from home, learn scripts overnight, work with different crews each day, deliver great work, and operate in a highly pressurized environment. My child's world had completely changed, and they were now speed-evolving to keep up. We have found that if you meet a child at their point of need, they – and their lives – will begin to change.

Child 3

Ch3 hilarious, wonderfully sarcastic, a great writer, creative, artistic, and has perfect pitch and a wild imagination. This is where they will find their purpose.

Every child is different

If you were to meet this child, you may be aware that they are different sooner than you might when meeting my other children.

In many ways, this can be an advantage for them. They do not feel the need to "mask" their autism or anxiety. In fact, they seem to have no choice in the matter, so they are simply themselves, showing up exactly as they are. They stim quite a bit, including pacing a lot. They are now in an autism school where they are among others who stim, and we have noticed their stimming has increased. In fact, Ch2 has noticed the increased stimming in their younger sibling, and started to stim as well, in order to help them with their anxiety.

Stimming can be an incredibly beneficial behaviour in both adults and children, helping to self-regulate sensation and feelings, but it can also look very obviously "different". Because of this, and because of a lack of understanding, stimming is one of the behaviours that neurotypical adults have tried to stop autistic children from doing. For some reason, it is considered socially unacceptable to move around in a way that is different from others, or to make sounds that others are not making. Have we never considered other people may benefit from doing the same – autistic or not? Every child is different – and for some, stimming will be a valuable part of the plan.

In addition to noticeable stimming, Ch3 has high levels of demand avoidance in their autism profile. PDA is sometimes talked about as a separate condition to autism, but it can also be seen as a trait within the autism spectrum, and it is increasingly being described as extreme demand avoidance (EDA) as opposed to the stigmatizing label "pathological". Here's the way it plays out in Ch3: they have an anxiety-led need to control situations, which presents in defiant behaviours. From the outside, it may look like a "naughty" child or just bad parenting – but believe me, this is not something that Ch3 would choose. "Getting their own way" is not the point, and often it is not how it works out at all – for example, Ch3 is excitedly looking forward to some wonderful event they have planned, but because they are asked to put their shoes and socks on, this sets off the anxiety-led need to feel in control … they then can't go. They are stuck – they want to do the "right" thing, and want to enjoy the event – but the need to feel safe and in control is stronger.

The way we have worked with this is to negotiate; we negotiate *everything*. Allowing Ch3 to feel as though they are controlling their life really helps but, as you can imagine, it goes against almost every parenting methodology out there, and it raises other issues around boundaries. Because, of course, there can also be times when Ch3's need for control spills over into other people's lives, situations, and environments. Obviously, no one grows up completely alone, so compromise will always be a part of our existence – but in our family, compromise can trigger anxiety or outbursts. We have found negotiation to be the best solution. So what does this look like in practice?

Here's an example. I do not tell Ch3 to get ready for bed, I just put two pairs of pyjamas on the end of the bed and say, "I wasn't sure if you'd prefer the blue or the green" and leave it at that. Sometimes this results in Ch3 getting ready for bed … and at other times I come in the next morning to find them in bed, still dressed in the school uniform from the night before. But I don't count this as a failure. How my children dress for bed does not matter in the grand scheme of things; these are low-priority issues. In my world, I am overjoyed that they went to bed and got some rest, or went to school, or ate dinner. I celebrate every good thing, and focus on what matters.

It's not always simple, of course. Negotiating can be a minefield, and with Ch3 in particular, if the adults allow something one day it is immediately, in their head, set in stone as a rule. One must be very canny. Plus there are other ways that a need to control can be very difficult for the child; if not channelled effectively, it can lead to other serious mental health issues such as obsessive-compulsive behaviours, disordered eating or finding our teens attempting to live alone in their very disordered, messy bedrooms. Staying actively engaged is super important – working with and around the difference, rather than fighting against it.

***

Autism =/= learning disability

There is another common assumption that people make about my children, which highlights the need to remember that every child – and every child with SEND – is different. Because Ch3 behaves or seems "more autistic", they are assumed to be more likely to have a learning disability. In fact, Ch3 is very bright and intelligent with no learning disability at all. Ch2 has dyscalculia, a learning disability that affects numbers (sort of how dyslexia affects letters and words) – they are effectively number blind, and at the age of 20 still struggle to tell the time. However, Ch3 has no such challenges. Then, all of my children – the ones with learning disabilities and those without, those with autism and those without – have vocabularies way beyond their years. It is important that we understand where there are strengths in each individual, and don't just assume challenges when they are not present.

***

Every child is evolving

When Ch3 was 11 years old and still in primary school, they began to feel very uncomfortable in their body and uncertain of their gender. They had started their period at the age of ten and, as with many autistic girls and those assigned female at birth, it was quite traumatic for them. Suddenly trying to navigate the adult world was a challenge, especially with the practical problem of there being no period facilities in the girls' toilets at school at the time. For Ch3, having to use the staff toilets was very stressful. So perhaps it makes sense that one day, when the whole family was gathered in our kitchen, Ch3 announced, "I am now a boy and I wish to be known as Ian."

Their two older siblings, horrified, immediately jumped in, saying, "No! Not *Ian*. That's a dreadful name!!"

I am so proud of this family moment. No one batted an eyelid about the idea of Ch3 transitioning; it was really just about the name they chose! Of course, there was more to it than the humour. I wanted to delve deeper with my child and find out the drivers for change – to learn about what was motivating them and also help them to understand what they might be facing. Over a two-year period, we had multiple conversations about their identity. David and I told them we would support them 100 per cent, whoever they were. And it wasn't just the gender dysphoria and struggles with puberty; I noticed that this was the time in school where they really began to recognize that they were different from the other children. All the children were going into a couple of the local secondary schools, but my child would be going to an autism school. I think they really found it hard that, after all these years, they would be separated from everyone and everything they had known at school up to that point.

One day I asked them a question.

"You do know that if you are a boy, you will still be an *autistic* boy, right?"

It was a moment of revelation for them, as they were confronted with the truth that they would always be autistic. Strangely enough, though, it was also the beginning of their absolute acceptance of being autistic. I don't want to pretend that this was some kind of magic proxy bullet for gender dysphoria or gender questioning – I'm not trying to say that all those who question their gender are actually just transferring feelings from something else. Having accepted their autistic identity, Ch3 continues to work through their identity as a whole: they have a wonderful, strong punk-indie image; they are a lesbian; they have very definite musical tastes. Lots of it is pretty concrete at this stage, but they continue to be very fluid with their gender.

What I am saying again with this story is that every child is constantly evolving, in big ways and small ways, and we are simply there to walk alongside, to listen, and to help when asked. People who have an agenda to change a child's decisions about their identity need to be very careful: our judgements, however subtle, will alienate the child. Focusing on trying to change a child's identity rather than changing the plan to accommodate the child can cause serious repercussions for their mental health, up to and including suicide. All young people, especially those with SEND, need time to work stuff out, and they will often benefit from talking to professionals who really understand the subject, especially for something as personal and tricky as gender dysphoria. The evolution between early childhood and adulthood can be a rocky road for all – we know, because we've all been through it! – and we need to give space and time to allow the full journey to take place.

The world is continually evolving

Ch3's world was upturned when they lost their place in the first autism school. Just at the point when they were struggling to work out why they had to separate from primary school, with all their neurotypical childhood friends, they were then told they didn't fit into an autism school either. They had a dawning realization that perhaps they didn't fit anywhere. This came at the exact age when they were working through their identity. It was devastating.

The Local Authority has a home tutoring service and sent a lovely lady to work with Ch3, but Ch3 but would not leave their bedroom and refused to talk to or interact with the teacher. It was also during this period that Ch2 had the TA coming into the home, and Ch4 had daily home visits from teachers as he transitioned into a new school. By default, and very much against our wishes, we had become home schoolers (long before COVID-19 made it a widespread necessity!). I spoke with my Local Authority, and the same amazing contact who made Ch2's school listen to us put me in touch with the autism head for the borough – an incredible woman who was full of compassion and creativity. She suggested we hold a meeting in the home with Ch3 and find out what they would like to do. Remember the demand avoidance? Suddenly, with this approach, Ch3 was in control. I prepared a list of about 100 activities, and Ch3 went through them all, ticking the ones they liked the sound of. It was negotiated and decided in this meeting that mornings would be time for a TA to come to the home and work with Ch3, including maths, English, and science. In the afternoons they would do drama, dog training, art class, piano, and, once a week, a trip out with two TAs. The new TAs were deliberately chosen: they were young, very cool, and with just the right attitude for Ch3. This curriculum was called an interim solution until another alternative school provision could be found. It went on for three years.

Ch3 had post-traumatic stress disorder (PTSD) levels of trauma from their autism school experience, so getting them to interact with the home-schooling, even though they had co-created it, was very challenging. Some days they wouldn't get out of bed; some days they were up, but very slow to get out of the house if it was an activity in another location. It became pretty much impossible for my husband and I to work, with TAs coming into the home, children having mental health breakdowns and everything else. By default, we halved our workload across our jobs and where we had previously worked together, this was now impossible. We have the privilege of having very good, very flexible jobs, though, so somehow we have worked things out. It is not the same for most other parents. Being able to get out of the house and get away from the situation was essential for our mental health. When I take a day out and make a TV programme, I come home feeling as if I've conquered the world. Being able to achieve the success of completing a task feels great. When we are in it for the long-haul, small wins matter – especially as our worlds are constantly changing.

Then the COVID-19 pandemic struck, we went into lockdown, and suddenly everyone's world changed. Lockdown was a very revealing time. Without the outside world being a part of our lives, our little nuclear family thrived. No judgement, no demands, no expectations. Each person was able to do as they pleased, interacting well with one another, anxiety lowered. Any issues we had actually arose as we *emerged* from lockdown, with the thought of returning to "life as normal".

It was during lockdown that I received a text from a friend who is the head of an autism school, letting me know a place had become available in Year 10 at their new upper school site. This school was one I had visited when Ch3 was first permanently excluded from the previous school. At the time it was in a different building, and the school didn't feel like a right fit for them for a variety of reasons. Once lockdown eased, Ch3 and I went to visit the new site and it was incredible: based in woodland, it is a great environment in which to learn. I loved the school ethos, how laid back everyone was, and how unflustered by some of the things I mentioned as potential issues. The most important indicator that we may have found the right school was that Ch3 walked in and said, "I want to come to this school."

I cannot overstate how miraculous this announcement felt to us as parents. During those three years of home-schooling, Ch3 had started to disassociate at the mention of the word "school". Staring into the distance, they would freeze, unable to move or sometimes even speak. If they did speak, it would be in the third person, talking as another character about themselves, and letting us know that Ch3 was not speaking to us. Sometimes, they would scream and swear and blame me for sending them to the first autism school, where they were left all day in one room alone with a teacher. The shouting was tolerable, if unpleasant – to be honest, I feel like their rage was valid, and I would often apologize to them for fighting to get them into a school that so traumatized them – but the disassociation was frightening. Soon they could no longer control when it happened to them; then it was happening daily and nightly. There have been many times when we were asleep and Ch3 would come in, begin shouting and throwing things, then suddenly disassociate. Having walked one child through suicidal ideation, I realized we were yet again staring a mental health breakdown in the face. Each August that Ch3 was out of school, just before the new school year began, they would put on their entire uniform from their old school and tell us that they were ready to go back, now. I would have to explain to them that there would be no going back: the exclusion was permanent. They knew this, but they wanted to let us know how they felt. All behaviour is communication, and they were letting us know exactly what was going on in their heart and mind.

So from this context the words "I want to come to this school" both delighted and terrified me. The child that had left the old school three years before was not the same child now; their world had drastically changed, multiple times. Isolation had changed them. Waiting for a school had changed them. Would the school understand my child's needs? Would the school cope with the dissociative episodes? And my biggest fear – what would happen if it went wrong again? I really felt that my child's life was at stake here.

In 2020, in the middle of the COVID-19 pandemic, my child went back to school. The first day we arrived, we were all wearing face masks, all students were in the new wooded outdoors area, and we spotted the head teacher of the upper school who Ch3 had not met before. Ch3 went marching up to them and said, "Can I get my nose pierced and still come to this school?"

It was a make-or-break moment. I knew that this was some kind of initiation test from Ch3. Slowly the head lowered her mask, revealing her whole face, and said, "Well, I have mine pierced, so I don't see why not."

I could have hugged that head. She knew exactly what my child was asking. It was about so much more than piercings.

Now, at the time of writing, they have been in the school for over a year and they are flourishing. The school is patient, full of strategies, and support – strategies that meet Ch3 in their difference, respond to them as they change and evolve, and take account of the changing world.

Child 4

Ch4 is sweet-natured, kind, helpful, loves animals, is good at debating and incredible at building and fixing things. Their purpose will be found in something that brings some or all of these areas together.

Every child is different

Ch4 is very different from my other children – of course, they are all different from each other, but the others have some things in common that Ch4 does not. The biggest difference I see is that he doesn't have the inner scaffolding of security that my other children have developed from birth – even through their worst struggles. Ch4's early life experiences left him with the belief that all things will end; he lives with the constant threat of abandonment. Try as we may to build a new scaffold and shoehorn it into him, realistically this has not been possible. He must live a life of faith that today is enough, and that we are here with him. This is not easy for him.

When he came to us, at the age of two, a simple request to eat his vegetables could result in an explosion. He would take sweets and hide behind the sofa. If I found him and said nothing other than to ask how he was feeling, he would explode. Predicting failure and loss, in his mind he wanted to explode his life before I had a chance to do it. By nature, Ch4 is very gentle and kind, and I have often thought that perhaps his violence comes from a need to protect or kick against that natural gentleness, because it makes him vulnerable.

Ch4 finds it almost impossible to make decisions. Decisions have been made about and for him his entire life. He has had no say, no power, no agency. Decisions, to him, can be catastrophic; one wrong move could lead to devastating consequences. The stakes are so high that he lives in a state of constant hypervigilance. When he came to us, he would sit in his high-chair and I would ask him what he wanted for breakfast.

"Rice Krispies," he would say.

I would pass him a bowl of Rice Krispies.

"No want it!" he would shout.

Gently, I would ask, "What would you like instead, Ch4?"

"Cornflakes."

I would pour the Rice Krispies back into the box and pour out some cornflakes. Passing them to him, he would shout,

"No want it!"

"What would you like, Ch4?"

"Rice Krispies."

This breakfast choice could cycle round for a long time. Sometimes, I would surprise him with another option or even simply take him out of the chair and tell him to let me know when he was ready to eat. But this didn't always work, either; Ch4 could bide his time, sometimes for *hours*. We would reach stalemate over and over again, over the choice of breakfast food, or anything and everything. Sometimes I would try to outsmart him. With my inner voice saying, "You will not beat me," I would leave some carrot and cucumber sticks on a low-lying table. I thought I was allowing him to have the control he needed, like leaving the choice of pyjamas out for Ch3. But Ch4 is not Ch3 – they are different, and their minds work differently, and their needs are different. I would return only to find the cucumber smeared all over the sofas and the carrot sticks in a hundred tiny pieces, chewed up and spat out.

Sometimes, I would try to go for the root issue and say, "You look like you need a hug. I'm just going to sit here on the floor, and you can come to me if you want." With a sense of defeat, he would retreat to the opposite side of the room. I would stay put. Then he would throw things at me, but I would stay sitting, silently telling him that I was not going anywhere. We would sometimes be held in a stalemate like this for up to an hour. I would wait patiently while he worked out how to get himself over to me for that hug. Eventually, exhausted, he would reverse into me, up into my lap and I would feel the tension leave his body. Then he would eat whatever I gave him.

Parenting or working with children takes time, and it's hard when you are in a situation like this and you have other children and work to do … but this is the joy of children. They are all different, and discovering who they are, and how they work, and whether and where you can influence their growth and happiness, is what makes it all worthwhile.

Every child is evolving

It took Ch4 a long time to attach to me – a very long time. He would attach to other women who came into his life, but resisted me for as long as he could hold out. In and out of school, he would spot any female adult (especially those with their own attachment issues) and before we knew it that person would become very mother-like to him. Everywhere he went he was looking for "Mum". This made my job much harder. Alongside this was another fear response: the fawn. He would tell me he loved me over and over – but there was no emotional resonance to it. It was a checking strategy, just to see if I was still present and secure. By the age of five (three years in), he began to be kinder towards me and more willing to chat and play with me. At seven, he stopped hitting me, and by eight he was holding me with sincerity and security.

Growing trust was *so hard* for Ch4. If he hurt himself, instead of seeking comfort he would run away and hide. Filled with shame, he would try his very hardest not to cry. I longed to be there for my child in these moments, but if I approached him he would scream at me. Another couple of years went by and he began to reverse into me for a backwards hug if he was hurt, and at the age of nine, he fully cried with me for the first time. With tears of vulnerability rolling down his beautiful cheeks, he looked me in the eye and trusted me with his pain. I will treasure this moment forever – not for his pain, of course, but because he finally felt safe and secure enough to allow me to *see* his pain. These days, I make sure to notice every lip tremble, every sign of vulnerability – not necessarily by pointing it out, but by making sure I am fully present and available in those moments.

The world is continually evolving

The effects of the COVID-19 pandemic have been both a blessing and a challenge for Ch4. He loved the security of everyone being at home together; it gave him a chance to fully cement his sense of family. Our family has a very strong sense of identity, and he now fully takes up his one-sixth of that identity. He now shapes the family as much as anyone else. There is a sense of ownership and belonging, and it has been beautiful to watch.

Perhaps growing from this deeper sense of security and belonging, it is also in this period that he expressed a desire to see his birth mother and half-brother. Every adoption story is different; in Ch4's case, I have been able to build a relationship with his "Tummy Mummy" over a number of years, behind the scenes, via text messages. Separately from Ch4, we have met up on neutral ground. We get on really well, and have a strong mutual respect for one another. She is now mum to a second child, and she is a great mum. For her, it's a success story – but adoption is complex and, as you can imagine, it may not be viewed in that way by my son. Before they met, I worried about how he would process his birth mother having another son and keeping him. What message would this give to my son? It's complicated, and I hate the fact that the adopted child has to do so much of the mental and emotional heavy lifting. But Ch4 had asked to meet them, so it was arranged. On the day, Ch4 was amazing: he was very real, casual yet curious, and very comfortable. Afterwards, he said, "I don't know why I've been putting that off for so long, it was great!" Fortunately, him meeting his "Tummy Mummy" has had no impact on our relationship; he is now secure in the knowledge that I am his Forever Mummy. He adapted so well to this world-changing lockdown, and even better to the world-changing meeting.

So that was lockdown; then came "back to school" and his young world changed yet again. At the time of writing, it has been a *nightmare*. In a constant state of hypervigilance, Ch4 has been in fight or flight mode for a whole year. Every few weeks, we have a serious incident at school.

When a child doesn't fit into – or is no longer welcome in – a mainstream school in the United Kingdom, they may end up in an AP (Alternative Provision) setting, or maybe in a PRU (Pupil Referral Unit). APs are designed to provide:

- education for pupils who, because of exclusion, illness, or other reasons, would not otherwise receive suitable education – decided by the Local Authority;
- education for pupils on a fixed-period exclusion from mainstream school – decided by the mainstream school;
- education for pupils to improve their behaviour off-site from mainstream school – decided by the mainstream school.

As you can see, for mainstream schools, an AP is seen as a short-term provision. Within the AP system are also PRUs. A child can end up in these schools when mainstream school isn't working for the child. I use the term "end up" here because, while many AP schools might be seen as a preferable alterative to mainstream school for some parents and young people, no parent would choose to take their child out of mainstream school for a PRU. Placements in PRU schools are decided by the Local Authority, and are usually longer term than many other AP provisions. (There is something of a movement to change this attitude;

some institutions have changed the acronym to mean Pupil Reintegration Unit, to give a sense of a plan for the child returning to mainstream school.)

Ch4 was sent to a PRU at the age of seven. I felt as if we had descended into hell; despite the resources and the amazing, incredibly highly trained staff, it still seemed like complete chaos to me. Eighteen children in three classes, with almost the same number of adults, there were calm-down rooms, therapy rooms, padded walled rooms – it was a whole new world. Even with therapists on site, and an attached hospital, I have been into the school hundreds of times over the years and not once have I found it at peace. There will always be a child in a corridor swearing and shouting at the top of their voice, making threats to kill or harm themselves or others, with one or more members of staff nearby. The atmosphere is traumatic for an adult visitor … let alone a child.

It's not all bad, though – every child is allocated a psychotherapist who works with both the child and the family on a regular basis, in a true attempt to make a plan that evolves with the child, meets them in their difference, and evolves as the world changes. The collaboration in this place, which has such an upsetting atmosphere, has been better than I have experienced in any other mainstream school.

However, collaboration wasn't enough at first to hit on the right strategy for Ch4. It is in this school, with its amazing staff, traumatizing and chaotic atmosphere, desire to collaborate, and children with extremely high support needs, that my child has punched, kicked, bitten, and thrown things at staff. It is here that he has trashed his classroom, upturned tables, broken countless windows, and smashed school equipment and staff property. It is here he has climbed onto the roof, scaled the scaffolding of the building next door, and absconded, being declared missing for hours while roaming around London alone. Police, ambulance, emergency helicopters, hospital-checks for staff – we've seen it all. And yet, in that same four-year period, he has been an angel at home. Something is clearly not working!

What changed Ch4's world at home was the moment we started practising non-violent resistance (NVR) – we'll look at this in more depth in the next chapter. At school, even with all the incredible expertise available, he continued to be very challenging. He spends every day of his school life in a state of fear. He is a very frightened little boy, scared of everything outside of his home. His response to this is fight or flight: he's either punching his way out or running. The most recent incident has meant his current PRU school no longer feels it is the right option for him. It feels as though he has been expelled from the last chance saloon. Where do we go now? My child needs an education. My child needs socialization. My child needs to feel safe and learn to operate well in society. And with the violence having no outlet at school, what will happen at home?

From my point of view, Ch4 needs a gentle school with a calm environment. Where is the school that is at peace, who can take my very dysregulated and un-peaceful child, and help him to settle? I'm not sure it exists … but I'm looking for it. There is a conundrum here. I would suggest that perhaps what most of these dysregulated children need is a very low-stimulation environment, and by default they all get sent to the same school where it's very difficult not to bounce off one another's dysregulation. Ch4's world has changed yet again – and we are still trying to work out how to adapt the strategy this time.

Behaviours that challenge

Before we move onto practical strategy, we should first think about the term "challenging behaviours" or "behaviours that challenge". This term is used to describe a whole range of behaviours, from violence to stimming, daydreaming to destruction of property. The question I always want to ask is this: challenge *who*?

When making a plan, this is a good place to start our thinking. The aim of parenting or teaching should not be to get people to do things *we* want, or to be able to tick off an arbitrary list of good actions; it should be to immerse the child in an atmosphere of good learning, guidance, and purpose. It is personal. It is about us discovering who this child is and why they are here. We are not here to make automatons; we are here to guide, teach, and encourage young humans in their humanity.

All behaviour is communication. All actions are telling us something. We may not like those actions, we may wish to stop those actions, but ultimately, if we are seeking change and development, we need to ask ourselves, "What is this child trying to tell me and how can I help?"

Learning objective: Parental toolkit

To equip yourself with various practical tools, techniques, and approaches that might make up part of a child's education strategy, including considering reasonable adjustments, and to begin to think creatively around strategies and adjustments that can be made.

5
Strategy
Tools, techniques, and tips

So, now we have the background, it's time to think about actually making the plan, choosing the elements that will make up the strategy for each individual. Over the years, we have found hundreds of strategies that have worked for our family. Some techniques have worked to varying degrees, or only worked for a particular period of time in our children's lives, and others have really stuck.

One thing worth pointing out is that we have learned to be magpies of all that is good. We don't want to rely on one source of ideas or stick religiously to one "methodology" – we are always actively seeking new ideas. I always say I hate going into meetings and being the most expert person present! I want to find those people who know the "deeper magic"; the people who have applied and adapted ideas in a number of ways, over a number of years, and with a number of different types of children. If you find someone with this breadth and depth of experience, try to get as many ideas from them as you can!

Non-violent resistance (NVR)

Earlier in the book, I mentioned a parenting style we have applied called non-violent resistance (NVR). NVR has its roots in the civil rights movement and was developed in Israel by Haim Omer (2004).

I will not cover the whole strategy here, but I will describe what we have used, what has worked for us, and how we have adapted the approach to work with autistic children and those with mental health challenges. The beauty of NVR is that it can – and should – be adapted and finely tuned for every situation. Remember, every child is different, every child is evolving, and the world is continuously evolving too. If you are an NVR practitioner, you may have done things differently to the way I will describe here, and that's just fine. What follows is how we made it work in *our* family, with *our* children.

NVR step 1: De-escalation

The first thing we learned was how to de-escalate a situation. With Ch4 increasingly expressing his needs and pain through violence, we desperately needed to understand how to bring down the temperature of a confrontation. Through working with an excellent trauma therapist, who was teaching us the NVR principles, we learned:

- There is no point trying to tell someone what they are doing wrong when they are in a rage or meltdown. They won't be able to hear you.
- A meltdown is also not the time to try to teach a child our parenting principles – again, they won't be able to take it in.

- It's not a win/lose binary. Either we all win or we all lose: if the rage/meltdown calms down, then we have all won, full stop.
- *Safety for all is a priority.*
- No matter how violent a child becomes, we (the parents/carers/professionals) do not use violence to control the situation. This is the *very core basis of NVR*. Refusing to meet violence with violence includes all forms of violent behaviour, not just physical – so that includes physical acts such as spanking or hitting, but also verbal and emotional violence such as shouting, intimidating, and so on.
- In the middle of a situation is not the time to apply punishments or threats. Even if they're non-violent punishments, the child will not be able to take it in; they are not responding with their rational minds right now, so punishments or threats are unlikely to work.

When we began to use this technique, we saw immediate change. Suddenly, Ch4 had nothing to bash up against in his meltdowns. Outbursts calmed down much more quickly, they were fewer in number, and they could be intercepted earlier. We began to more clearly recognize the build-up and the triggers, and we could step in a lot sooner. It didn't always work – but over time, with consistent use, we began to see great change.

This kind of de-escalation is not only useful for child-on-parent violence. Ch4 can also get into a state where he experiences a sense of omnipotence and can display very dangerous actions. I remember one time when the building behind his school had been gutted by a fire and was surrounded by scaffolding. Somehow, my son managed to climb up onto the rear wall of the school and up onto the scaffold. He then proceeded to climb up two storeys to a very dangerous height and threatened to climb into the burned-out house. This action would have meant almost certain death for Ch4: the whole building was unstable, with no proper functioning floors left. The police, ambulance, and fire services were called. Far from being afraid, though, in that moment my son was empowered. There was not one scintilla of fear in him.

De-escalation in those situations is vital. In our case, the police eventually talked him down safely. From this, we learned to ask questions around the connection between abject fear of learning for Ch4 and the absolute empowerment that he found in danger. If there is a benefit to escalation, then a child will push in that direction. In Ch4's case, he was clearly finding a sense of control in escalating dangerous situations, so for de-escalation to work, we have to help him to find some sense of control in a safer way.

Meltdowns versus tantrums

It is important to note that there is a difference between a meltdown and a tantrum. They can look very similar, and it can be tempting to simply believe that you should never give into a child's tantrum for fear of spoiling them. But they really are different experiences – with a tantrum, the child is still pretty much in conscious control of their behaviour. A tantrum may pass in ten minutes or so, whereas a meltdown can last for an hour or more. Meltdowns happen when a child loses control, becomes overwhelmed by what they are experiencing, and lacks the ability – for whatever reason – to express themselves other than to simply melt down into rage, terror, anguish, or violence.

A tantrum might stop if you offer a bribe, like sweets or an ice cream – whereas trying to bribe your way out of a meltdown will be unsuccessful because the child has simply lost the ability to regulate themselves.

De-escalation (like a lot of NVR techniques) can be used for both tantrums and meltdowns – it is not "giving in to a tantrum" but rather refusing to meet violence with violence, and drawing the heat out of a situation until it can be constructively dealt with. It might be tempting to ask how, if a child is always pandered to, he actually learns anything – but the key is that NVR doesn't end at de-escalation. One part is non-violence, and the other part is *resistance*. Instead of reacting in the moment, you have to deal with it when everyone is able to deal with it – you have to strike while the iron is cold.

NVR step 2: Strike while the iron is cold

Once calm has resumed, we wait for the right moment to discuss what happened. Sometimes it's half an hour later, sometimes it's a day later. Timing is crucial: too early and we can find ourselves back facing the rage. Acting when things are calm is by far the better way of unpacking and discussing behaviours that challenge. In the calm, we can think, our child can reflect, and we can all take responsibility for the moments where we know we have done or said something wrong. When we are calm, we can find a place of agreement, we can negotiate, we can correct, we can say sorry, and we can use these situations to make good bonds. None of this can happen in the heat of the moment!

Remember: all behaviour is communication. Meltdowns happen when a child runs out of ways to express something – even tantrums are a way of communicating something. If you have had a rage or a tantrum, it may not have been very sophisticated, but something was happening for the child. What is this child trying to tell us? Most of the time, at the root of the issue, our children are telling us:

- I hate myself.
- I hate my life.
- I am hurting.
- I'm scared.
- You won't let me have or do something I want to have or do.
- You have made a demand I cannot fulfil.

Sometimes my children seem to have a mixture of all of the above, so there's a lot to unpick – and clearly, it helps for everyone to be calm while we try and work through those beliefs and feelings.

NVR step 3: Top-box priority

This is one of my very favourite parts of NVR. Similar to how de-escalation prioritizes safety and calmness before trying to tackle to root of an issue, the top-box technique is a way of prioritizing the behaviours we are encountering. When we are struggling with our children, it sometimes feels as though everything is wrong and we do not even know where to begin. I used to joke with Ch1, "Give me something to work with!"

So, when everyone is calm, we sort a child's problematic behaviours into three sections:

1. *The middle box:* The first thing we do is to assess the behaviours that are really challenging, the stuff that really

matters, the "deal-breakers" that have to be addressed. This list (and sometimes it is a list) goes into the middle box.

2. *The bottom box:* This is the stuff that is unimportant in the grand scheme of things. We don't sweat the small stuff.

3. *The top box:* At this point, we go back to the middle box and choose the one behaviour on which we are going to focus. This may be something smallish for an easier win, or a big challenge, depending on what we feel we or our child can cope with.

This model gives parents, professionals, and teachers – and young people – a sense of direction. While using this tool, it's important to remember that we are not just setting out to change behaviours we find challenging; we are trying to understand our children in depth, to really get what is happening for them. This isn't operant conditioning – we don't want to simply force a child to abandon a behaviour that is serving to communicate something for them. Rather, we want to understand what it is that the child is trying to communicate with this behaviour

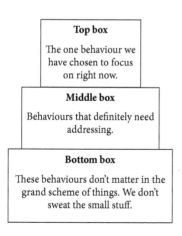

Figure 7 Behaviour boxes

– consciously or unconsciously – and work with them to find a safer and more effective way to communicate that thing. The way we do that is through two other NVR tools.

NVR step 4: The announcement

When we first looked at the top-box model it was with Ch4 in mind.

1.   *The middle box:* We had physical violence towards adults, physical violence towards other children, swearing, smashing property, slamming doors, shouting, growling, spitting, throwing things, and weeing on the floor.

2.   *The bottom box:* We had refusal to eat, eating until he threw up, breaking toys, ignoring people, refusing to join in activities, and laying on the ground when asked to move.

3.   *The top box:* We started with "weeing on the floor", as we felt this may be easier to tackle than some of the other behaviours. Ch4 was nearly five years old. He would go into a room, urinate on the floor, then walk away. He was totally toilet trained, so we knew it was an intentional action.

In the past, to try to tackle this behaviour, I had:

1.   raised my voice and sent him to the naughty step;

2.   raised my voice and sent him to sit on his bed for five minutes;

3.   told him he had to clear the wee up and handed him some kitchen towels; and

4.   tried to out-psych him by cleaning it up and saying nothing.

Nothing worked. Still he persisted with this behaviour.

This is the next part of the work – the resistance part, the find-a-better-way part. Ch4's fear of abandonment and shame had him performing some strange behaviours. For him, urinating on the floor was a compulsion strongly related to those feelings of shame and fear of abandonment; the action compounded those feelings, but he couldn't stop doing it because it was serving a need for control over those feelings. So, instead of punishing, we used the top-box method to choose this one behaviour to focus on, and then used the next step – the announcement – to try to provide Ch4 with a more helpful and effective way of tackling those feelings.

The announcement is written down – it should have a certain sense of ceremony or formality about it. In this case, it looked something like this:

> Ch4, you are an amazing child, and you are loved and so valuable to our family. We all love you and appreciate all you bring into the family. We have noticed you have been weeing on the floor and we would like you to stop doing this. We are totally committed to helping you with this, so we are going to come up with some ideas together. Thank you for listening. Love Mummy and Daddy.

Back then, Ch4 couldn't read, but we wrote it down anyway, sat down together, read it to him, and gave him a copy. He listened, made no visible response and at the end of it walked off with the announcement in his hand.

We were ready for a lot more work – we were prepared to go on to the next step, the sit-in, but sometimes simply making the announcement is enough. Perhaps it was the way we formally communicated love and acceptance to give Ch4 a slightly increased sense of security; perhaps it was that we tackled the issue face-on, without judgement or shame – but whatever it was, from that day to this, he has never intentionally urinated on the floor. Clearly, approaching him in this way had a different impact from all our other strategies.

We were so shocked that we jumped straight in with a very big challenge: to stop hitting me. This one took a little longer, and we needed to call on the next step in the NVR toolbox.

NVR step 5: The sit-in

Having moved "hitting Mummy" into the top box, we delivered the new announcement. It was very similar to the first announcement, but in this case it replaced the sentence about weeing on the floor with:

> "You have been punching Mummy and you need to stop doing this."

And then we had our first "sit-in". This is an essential part of any civil rights movement: in social politics, it is often a declaration that you are not moving until something changes. In terms of working with children and young people, it takes the form of entering their space and asking them to work with you. It is not dissimilar to what I was doing instinctively when I would go to Ch4's room and hold the space, waiting for him to make a move – but in this case, it is specifically focused on all parties working together on the last part of the announcement:

> "We are totally committed to helping you with this, so
> we are going to come up with some ideas together."

In a moment where the iron was definitely cold, we entered our child's bedroom and sat down. David was silently supporting me while I spoke to Ch4 directly, with a kind tone:

> "We spoke to you about punching Mummy, and this
> is what happened again yesterday. So today we are
> going to think together about what we can do to stop
> this from happening."

It certainly wasn't a magic bullet. Hitting me had become a very deeply ingrained behaviour for Ch4, an expression of some of his deepest hurt. That first time, he threw every toy in his room at me. He threw until he was exhausted from throwing. Finally, when he tried to throw his bed mattress, I asked him to stop and we left the room – it is important to balance the sit-in with not overwhelming a child. If we had stayed then, it might have escalated into a meltdown – we must keep striking when the iron is cold.

A couple of days later, we did the same thing again. I repeated my statement that he had to come up with an idea we could work on.

This time, there was no throwing.

"I'm going to smash the whole house up," he declared through gritted teeth.

"This is not such a good idea, as then we won't have anywhere to live or sleep," I calmly replied.

We sat in silence.

A while later: "I'm going to go and live on the moon," he screamed.

I took a breath, "This is not such a good idea, as it's impossible to do. Perhaps you could be really clever and think up something that could work."

Silence.

A while later: "I'm going to go into the lounge and lay on the blue sofa."

"Yes!! Great idea."

We'd cracked it. *He'd* cracked it. He had come up with an idea. I was doubtful it would work, if I'm honest. Perhaps we were grasping at straws, and I didn't really think it was a great idea, but none of that mattered as much as this: we could immediately tell that he was seriously attempting to collaborate with us. That was the real win here – not his idea in and of itself, but that fact that he worked with us to come up with one. And to really cement how useful this tool was going to be for us, it turned out that, actually, his idea was a good one. Over the coming weeks, I saw my son laying on that sofa so many times until I realized that he was using this location to self-regulate. Far from being the dud that I had feared, it was actually a genius idea! Because he had chosen a certain space for himself, and decided to use it, and *how* to use it, he took complete ownership over his attempts to manage his own feelings and remove himself from situations that might otherwise escalate. Instead of us laying down the law and simply providing a wall for him to hit – physically and metaphorically – this tool enabled us to support Ch4 in maintaining his own healthy boundaries without violence. A few weeks later, the hitting had stopped.

I cannot overstate what a win this was for our family. Just imagine you visited my home around this time. We sit drinking tea, having a chat, when my son stands up, tells me to F-off, slams the kitchen door, and stomps upstairs. Perhaps shocked, perhaps offended, or perhaps sympathetic, you turn to me to commiserate or offer advice … only to then see David and I give each other a happy thumbs up. You'd probably think you'd entered topsy-turvy world! But in our world at that time, when this kind of thing happened, we were just so excited and grateful that he hadn't hit me. Seeing him find other ways of expressing his rage and pain was a massive win in our view. It was a family success. And on a side note, this experience has taught me to be less judgemental of other parents too – whenever I see how parents are working with their children, I remind myself that they may be intervening in a way I have no idea about.

The amazing part of life during this period was realizing we were back in control in terms of our parenting. We had felt so unable to parent, so defeated, failing at every turn. Before, we were either shouting or passively hiding. We couldn't find the middle ground. We had no idea what to do but this was an absolute breakthrough. These days, Ch4 still finds his way to that little blue sofa. He probably has no idea why it feels good to lie there.

Adapting tools for different needs

Adapting our parenting methods for different needs – specifically autism or mental health challenges – has been essential. Personally, we wouldn't use the announcement with our other children, but we have adapted the sit-in to good use.

When a child is depressed, has suicidal ideation, and is self-harming, the harmful behaviour is different from hitting out at others, but can still be tackled as a top box priority. With a couple of my children, I have skipped the formality of the Announcement and simply gone to sit in their bedroom.

With Ch2, the conversation went like this:

> "Why are you here?"
> "I thought I'd come and sit with you."
> "You're being weird. Can you get out?"
> "I will in two minutes."

They stare at the clock. Two minutes later:

> "Can you please leave now?"
> "Sure."

Two days later, I do the same again.

> "What are you doing here? Why are you doing this again?"
> "I'm just going to sit here for a few minutes."

We sit in hostile silence.

A couple of minutes later, I get up to leave, saying, "Thanks darling" as I go.

A few days later, I do the same thing again; this continues for a couple of weeks.

Over time, I increased the length of time I spent in Ch2's space. I was never there for more than about ten minutes, but I persisted, and after about two weeks Ch2 started speaking to me while I was there. They began to share how they were feeling. After another few weeks of this, they began to initiate, asking me to come to their room instead of waiting for me to turn up. Sometimes we would speak: occasionally it was about serious stuff, sometimes it was very casual. Often, it was simply my presence that helped to intercept the intrusive thoughts they were experiencing. Sometimes, when things were really tough, I simply shared the silence. It was both painful and magical.

This is an example of how a method can be shifted and adapted for different needs and situations. For Ch4, we needed him to take ownership of channelling his emotions in a way that was not violent towards me (or anyone else). It was passive, but still a confrontation – I won't move until you do this (come up with an idea). With Ch2, a confrontation would not have worked at all, but the idea of the physical presence and silent support that made up part of the approach with Ch4 was perfectly suited to Ch2's needs. With all these methods and tools, it comes back to the principles we explored in the last chapter – a strategy must be based on knowing the child and their needs. There is no one-size-fits-all approach.

NVR step 6: Consequences and gifts; punishments and rewards

Another NVR principle that we found incredibly helpful for our family was the idea of punishments and rewards. Before NVR, we had been falling back on the old "carrot-and-stick" approach that most everyone knows – reward good behaviour and punish bad. But, as you have seen, it wasn't working.

The first change in our approach came from teasing out the difference between consequences and punishments. It's quite simple, once you start thinking about it: consequences are going to happen irrespective of my actions as a parent, whereas a punishment is something I have to take action on. So a child climbing up the tree when they have been asked not to, then breaking their leg – well, now they have a broken leg. That's a consequence.

However, if I were to threaten my child with taking away their electronics because they were not putting them down during mealtimes or when they should be in the bath – that would be a punishment, because I have to take action for it to happen. Confusingly, some parenting methods would frame this latter punishment as a "consequence", which is understandable – a child needs to eat and be clean, so if they're refusing to do so because of using electronic devices, it seems like it would a natural consequence for those devices to be confiscated, right?

Except that it still takes an action on the adult's part. It's not a natural consequence to the child; they will see it as something I am actively doing to them. For a child with attachment issues or self-loathing, punishments and rewards are really unhelpful. Experiencing punishments, no matter how well-intentioned or how much love they are done with, can cause an increase in anxiety, leading them to shut down, feel shame, or push against the system – especially if they feel (rightly or wrongly) that they can never reach the bar the adult is setting; this only leads to despair and more self-hate. You might see this in reactionary behaviours such as them hitting out or self-harming in some way. This is because, for many children, punishment equals "you don't love me" or "I am no good". Reward equals "you love me" or "I am okay as long as I have this reward" – which is clearly an equally unhealthy thing to be inadvertently teaching our children. The concept of experiencing a negative action as an expression of love and care is a very difficult one for children to understand – and, to be honest, even for children who do manage to grasp the concept, it can then lead to issues later in life when they associate someone "punishing" them with love and care, so priming young adults to accept abuse in relationships. So, all in all, we needed to change the way we think about punishment and reward.

The NVR approach is to remove them altogether. I'll be honest: it was scary. We chose to go along with it, and at first it felt as if we had been completely disarmed in a battle. We were sure it would lead to us simply getting trampled, but soon enough we began to see the fruit. Our relationships with all the children improved. They grew in confidence and security in our love. We had always told them our love was unconditional, and now they could see for themselves that this was the case, as they did not have to earn rewards.

We still have strong boundaries, but the breaking of a boundary is now discussed and the motivation is explored. Sometimes, this leads to a boundary being renegotiated. We don't reward our children for following rules; instead, we thank them when they honour a boundary. We tell them how they are helping us all to grow in trust of one another. And they don't lose out on the gifts that rewards might otherwise have been; now we will sometimes leave little gifts out for them just because. They know they have not earned these gifts; they are there simply because we love them. They leave out little gifts for one another now too, with no strings attached – just because.

General tools, approaches, and strategies

As I mentioned at the start of this chapter, we have become magpies for good ideas, and not every tool that we use in our family comes from the NVR methodology. Here are some of the other strategies that work or have worked for us in different circumstances across different areas of life, and for different children.

Being present

The importance of being present cannot be under-estimated. It is less a discrete tool and more of an approach or attitude shift. It is one thing to be in the room geographically, but it is quite another to be present, in the moment, undistracted, and giving our full attention. It is not always easy: giving full attention to anything can be tiring, and if our children are challenging, it can sometimes feel like the opposite of what we need. I know that when I am exhausted, I am more likely to "check out" from the kids. It's a survival tactic, and sometimes a necessary one. I'm not saying we shouldn't ever check out as parents or carers; however, if and when we do so, we need to remain aware that it's best used as a temporary state. And this is most applicable to parent-carers who are around their children all the time – for professionals who usually have a set amount of contact time with children, it's even more crucial that they spend that time fully present and aware.

But it's not all hard work – being fully present can make some things easier. I found that the great thing about it is that it takes the pressure off having to say something, know all the answers, or come up with a solution. Because, let's be honest, adults don't know everything! Being present is to intentionally "hold the space". Our children are very aware when we do this, and it helps them to feel safe – often, much safer than if we fudge a vague answer that ignores their feelings, or pretend we know the answers when they can tell we don't. Don't under-estimate how effective this can be: there is something incredibly healing about another human sitting alongside us in our pain without trying to shift or change us. You might have experienced it yourself – think about how you feel, now, as an adult, when you express sadness or hurt to a friend or partner, and they immediately start giving advice about how you could do things differently. Or when they don't listen properly, or tell you you're probably overreacting. Now consider how you feel when you express hurt or sadness and your friend or partner listens to you – really listens – and gives you the space to feel what you're feeling safely, and to know that you are accepted and loved. It's no different for children.

Our children and young people are capable of great thinking, and will often find the answers to the issues they face if we allow them to discover what's going on within themselves. Our job as parents and teachers is to steer like a shepherd, using a metaphorical staff to gently guide. There is a time for everything, of course, and sometimes our young people will need carrying through a situation – but there is something incredible about a child learning the skills for themselves. We help them with this by creating these safe spaces and safe moments.

When we learn to "hold the space", we put the person (not ourselves) in the centre of the conversation or listening. We are slow to jump in; we are hearing and believing the person as they speak and allowing them to journey through an issue. This allows them to identify the story, to shape and change their thinking, and to create their own narrative. If you want to read more about holding space in this way, Professor Arietta Slade and Dr Jeree Pawl have written a lot on the subject – for example see Slade and Holmes (2013) *Attachment Theory* (6 vols) and Pawl and Dombro (2001) *Learning and Growing Together with Families: Partnering with Parents to Support Young Children's Development*.

Listening

This follows on from being present. Most of us know the importance of listening, but it's worth repeating, because it is crucial. And real listening is about more than our ears – it requires truly taking in what is being said and communicated, to inwardly assess what is going on. Sometimes talking is over-rated, especially for our children who have social communication differences, so one of my most worked-on skills has been to listen with everything I have – to focus on everything they are communicating, not just the words they might be saying or not saying. I use my ears, my eyes, my heart and mind, and my "felt space" – or what you might call gut or intuition. Once we begin to utilize all our senses, we see a lot more than we have before.

For example, I notice that my children's breathing is often laboured when they are stressed or anxious, which is one of the early signs that something may be bothering them. Words can be very confusing for both the speaker and the listener; sometimes when any of us are processing our thoughts, we don't always make sense. So how do we hear what's not being spoken? How do we become a good sounding board?

Slow down, empathize, repeat

When children are dysregulated, they often find it hard to produce the right words to express the level of emotion they are experiencing, or define exactly what caused the dysregulation.

When Ch1 is dysregulated, they experience very chaotic thinking. The hyperactive part of their ADHD is moving at 100 miles an hour, thoughts bounce around their head, and it becomes very hard for them to find what they want to say. Some of my other children also experience this; they may get very angry as a result of their frustrated communication, and things can escalate very quickly. Slowing the conversation down, giving space, and encouraging them to take their time really helps. Sometimes it's as simple as saying: "I am not going anywhere. I am here to listen and not judge."

At other times, though, my children need very little encouragement to keep speaking! What helps them along the road towards communicating effectively among the flow of words is to be met with the language of empathy. This might look like focusing on and holding eye contact with them while remaining verbally silent. Or I might simply nod, or give a "gosh", a "wow", a "that's hard", a "that must hurt" or "I hear you" – all words and phrases that let them know I hear them, believe them, understand.

Once I know they are past the first outpouring and they come to a natural pause, if it's appropriate I may then repeat what they have said back to them. Here's an example:

Child: The teacher hates me, and they don't want me in the class.

Me: I hear you: the teacher hates you and they don't want you in the class.

I am not agreeing or disagreeing. I am not passing judgement. I am simply choosing to hear my child. I cannot emphasize enough the importance of being heard without judgement. The whole world needs this right now! Too often, when we work with children, we try to solve their problems or invalidate what they are telling us. I could immediately try to refute what they're saying:

Me: That's not true – the teacher loves you.

But what effect would this have? My child would feel like I wasn't listening to them, and communication would stop. If we are to change anything, we must first hear what is being said. It is not actually relevant whether it is true or not; first and foremost, it's about hearing how the person is experiencing the world. Our children are not always looking for us to solve their problems. They are telling us they are hurt; that they feel angry or fearful or stupid or ashamed. How the words tip out makes no difference. Repeating back to them the words they have said helps the child to reflect and think about whether it rings true for them. Often, a child will then change what they say on the second attempt:

Child: I hate being in the class because I feel stupid.

Me: I hear you. You hate being in the class because you feel stupid.

Then, maybe, comes attempt number three:

Child: I didn't understand the maths. I can't do it.

Me: Okay. You didn't understand the maths. You can't do it.

I might then wait quietly – allowing the time and space to see whether anything more needs to be said. If it seems as if they are finished speaking, or they want some input from me, I might then think about offering a solution based on what they have told me:

Me: Sometimes maths is a nightmare. Would you like me to have a look at it with you?

Obviously, this example is a simplified version of events, but the principle remains true. Being heard is essential, and without first hearing what a child is saying, change cannot take hold.

"What" not "why"

We always ask our children *what* happened, not *why* it happened. The question "What?" is concrete; they can explain the details. "Why?" is problematic. When a child does something very extreme it's hard not to ask why – but children are not always able to access their motivation with any real clarity. (For that matter, we adults don't always know exactly why we do what we do!) Besides, what is a child really expected to say? What is an adopted child going to say when asked why they lashed out?

"Oh I did that because when I was a baby, this thing happened to me and …"

I cannot expect my child to psychoanalyse themselves to that level. How far are am I expecting them to go back? For me, focusing on what happened is much more constructive. The why might come out later as the conversation progresses – but in the initial ask, I focus on the what.

Shame

There is a little word I have mentioned here and there in passing throughout the stories in this book. It's a little word, but it has a gigantic impact: shame.

Shame as an emotion has no earthly use to the one who feels it. It is useful only to others as a manipulative tool to oppress and control; it will unravel our very identity and have us chasing our tails. Shame will lead us down the road of low self-esteem and set up home for us in an inner city of self-loathing. It leads to self-destructive behaviours and unhelpful drivers. I have never seen shame lead to anything good. Regret is helpful; remorse is helpful; understanding right from wrong, knowing where we have gone wrong and owning our mistakes are helpful – but none of this is the same as the absolute self-destruction that shame unleashes on us.

Helping our children to live lives free from shame surely has to be one of the most important aspects of living or working with children. The next time you use social media, notice how many times the phrase, "You should be ashamed of yourself!" is used by people who are grown adults. It's everywhere, and our children pick up on it – in social media but also in school, sadly, and sometimes even at home. Our children notice how we feel about ourselves and if we comment shamefully about ourselves. We model the good and bad of self-esteem.

Helping our child to turn the inner harsh, shaming judge into the good and fair judge is really important. It is one of the core values required as we teach our children to develop a healthy mindset. It declares, "You are enough." This can be seen in the NVR tools, for example – de-escalation and sit-ins both rely on an approach that does not cause a child to feel shamed but supported.

Sorry and forgiveness

Without shame, apologies and forgiveness suddenly become a lot more accessible.

As someone who never heard an apology growing up, I cannot tell you the depth or impact the word "sorry" carries for me. It is healing balm. It is redemption. It is freedom. When I first met my husband, he said sorry regularly when he did something wrong, and it would make me cry; I felt like I had waited so long just to hear someone say it. Gradually, I began to use the word myself – although it took practice!

A sincere "sorry" takes both parties to the roots of trust and to our perception of whether we lose or gain power. In our family, we have made sure to create an environment where we apologize when we hurt one other. We never apologize for our existence, or "over-sorry" at every juncture, but nor do we refuse to apologize out of a misguided sense of power, pride, or fear. When we hurt the people we love, it is only right that we let them know this wasn't what was meant to happen.

Note how I'm talking about this, too – as a consequence, not a goal. We have never made "saying sorry" a top-box behaviour, and we have never made apologizing a boundary or a rule. Rather, we have tried to create an environment where, without shame getting in the way, and with clear communication and genuine listening, an apology is the natural response when we hurt someone. A sorry should not be demanded of someone – it won't be genuine, and it won't work – but it can be demonstrated and set up to become a normal part of life.

An apology's greatest partner is forgiveness. Hear me out: I know this might be an old-fashioned word, perhaps with religious connotations that aren't necessarily helpful, but the concept has value. For example, I prefer to tell my children, "I forgive you," than "That's okay." Think about when I was dealing with Ch4's direct rage and violence towards me: it's not okay to punch me, and I would never want to teach him or tell him that it was. But I did, and do, choose to forgive him. It's important too to note that forgiveness, for our family, is not necessarily reliant on a genuine apology – in fact, sometimes the former comes before the latter. A sorry may not have been sincere, but explicit forgiveness nevertheless reinforces that sense of security, and demonstrates a shame- and judgement-free environment.

Self-care and supporters

This is an area we talked a lot about during our adoption training before adopting Ch4. It is the most overlooked area in our parenting lives, too. Sometimes it feels impossible to care for ourselves when we are in intense situations with our children. However, after lots of practice, I am now sure to let my children know when I need space, when I need to finish a task/have a bath/eat before I can assist them, or when I am going away overnight for some time with Dad. Things may kick off as a result, but we have to care for ourselves or there will be no family. This is true for all who care for children, in any capacity: teachers, social workers, health workers, whoever. It is essential that our needs are heard, and rest is had, otherwise our capacity to give care diminishes rapidly. In addition, taking care of ourselves is an important part of modelling a healthy life for our children. When you care for a child, especially a child with additional needs, it can be tempting to sacrifice everything – every moment of rest, every positive action for ourselves, every shower or meal – to taking care of them. But what does this teach them? That when they grow up, they will also have to ignore all their own needs? No – self-care matters.

And it doesn't have to be a solo journey. Caring for children with high needs can feel very isolating; as adults, where do we find supporters? I'm not going to pretend it's easy. In fact, we found it so difficult to find support that eight years ago we started a parent support group in our home, because we realized we knew no people in the same situation as ours. We started with about 10 parents, and to date the group has grown to over 170 families. For us, they are the best people to talk to about the challenges of parenting our amazing children, because they really get it. They understand the stresses we feel, and sharing is cathartic. But not everyone will have to start their own group; professionals should have systems set up to get support from managers or peers, and there are many parent/carer support groups around. The official ones can usually be found on the Local Authority website under "Local Offer". Similarly, in schools, forming small support groups can really help. There are many on different social media platforms.

Sensory integration

Every person processes life through their senses: they are the gateway to information going in, and the brain processes the input to help us understand what we are seeing, touching, hearing or feeling. If too much information is going in, the brain gets overloaded. The light becomes too bright, the noises too loud, the smells too strong, taste and touch become difficult. This will be more common in autistic people – especially autistic children, before they develop the coping mechanisms that might help them – but it's true for all children and adults. Everybody's capacity for dealing with sensory input is different, and if the person is trying to regulate all this input while also attempting to learn or interact socially, it becomes doubly hard.

Many years ago, I remember an expert in the field of sensory integration used the following example, with Winnie the Pooh as a metaphor. Some children wake up like Tigger: bouncing off walls and over-stimulated. In contrast, some children wake up like Eeyore: slow, very sensitive to touch and sound, and needing very gentle stimulation to wake fully. Interestingly, though, both states benefit from the same method to help the child to regulate the super-speedy or slow-paced senses: proprioceptive activity. This is a kind of activity that helps to regulate the senses and prolongs periods of concentration. Proprioceptive activities might include pushing and pulling or weight-bearing exercise; trampolining; chewing and sucking motions; and deep body pressure from hugs or a weighted blanket.

With all our children, we have noticed the impact of physical activity on concentration and emotional regulation. When put regularly into their daily routine at school, it has been incredibly beneficial.

Interoception

Interoception is another sense now being talked about more widely in our community. It is the perception of sensations from inside the body. Interoception includes the perception of physical sensations related to internal organ function such as heartbeat, respiration, and satiety, as well as the autonomic nervous system activity related to emotions (Barrett et al., 2004; Cameron, 2001; Craig, 2002; Vaitl, 1996). Interoception is also used for us to tell ourselves when we need the bathroom, or when we are in pain, or when we are hungry. When I first heard about this concept, it was a revelation to me: I had often pondered why my children hop from one foot to the other, needing to go to the loo but not going until they absolutely have to. Or why they might suddenly realize that they are desperately hungry, but there doesn't seem to be a lead-up to the desire to eat and we are faced with a "hangry" child!

It is worth developing our knowledge of the senses in ourselves and also noticing how the senses are impacting our children. Evidence suggests that neurodivergent people may struggle with interoception in the same way that they can struggle to regulate other sensory input – perhaps being less sensitive to interoception (as my children seem to be sometimes), or perhaps being more sensitive, like being unable to concentrate over the sensation of their own heartbeat. Maybe both tendencies could occur in the same person – the key, as we saw in Chapter 4, is to get to know the child with whom you are working and start to consider how they might experience sensory input, including interoception.

School-specific tools

Many of the tools in this chapter will work most effectively when used consistently across a child's life, from home to school and wherever else they might be. But school is such a significant part of any child's life – whether they are attending currently or not – that we have definitely found some tools and techniques that are specifically useful for a child's educational setting.

Factors that impact a child in school

With Ch2 and Ch3 in particular, I found that there were four questions that, when considered properly, made my children's lives (and their access to education) easier:

1.   What is the environment like?
2.   What is the child's relationship with the subject like?
3.   What is the child's relationship with the teacher like?
4.   What is the child's relationship with their peers like?

What is the environment like?

When I go into primary schools, I am still stunned by the sheer number of pieces of art hanging from the ceiling, the posters, and explosions of colour on every wall. While this is no doubt cheerful for some children, for many it will be incredibly distracting. I know that as an adult, if I am writing a song, I need to look at a blank wall – I need to regulate what can distract me, and focus on my creative output instead of the stimulation of art, colour, texture, and so on. I have no idea how children are supposed to create stories, use their imagination, or focus on learning with so much stimulation in front of them. A regulated sensory environment is best for all children, generally speaking – including neurotypical children or those without additional learning needs. Is the room too hot or too cold? If it's at the end of a corridor, is there a squeaky door just beside the classroom? Does the room smell bad? All these things can make life irritating for anybody, but can be really difficult for children with sensory sensitivities. It is also worth considering where the child sits in a classroom. They may need to sit closer to the front, to help them avoid the distractions of other students in front of them – but they may also hate this concept if they have issues with anxiety, so it's worth checking. Or maybe they need to be moved away from sources of heat or cold, or away from the speakers – and so on.

What is the child's relationship with the subject like?

We often found that while our children were in primary school, there would be particular days or times of day when they would struggle. This might have been to do with their own rhythms – for example, I'm sure we all recognize what it feels like to have a mid-afternoon slump! – but in the structured environment of primary school, it might also be a particular subject with which they struggle.

This is important to consider not just from a learning angle, but also from a fear angle. A child might not have difficulty with learning a topic; there might be something instead that's triggering fear, anxiety or sensory overload – for example, Ch2 struggled for a while with a fear of black and white photographs, so found history lessons at primary school really difficult. And it's not just primary school; there is often an over-emphasis on taking every subject at secondary school as a metric for achievement. But if a child is struggling with a particular subject – say, a language – why not drop that subject from their timetable? Dropping a subject almost never has a really significant negative impact on a child's overall academic attainment, and if it means the child remains in school, I would suggest that it's not something worth fighting over. If a child needs space for their mental health, this can be a great strategy to create "free" periods that can be spent in quiet, doing homework with support, or in sensory regulation.

What is the child's relationship with the teacher like?

This is absolutely crucial to any child. If a child knows the teacher doesn't like or is frustrated by them, they will act out accordingly – just as you and I might. Imagine spending all day, every day, with a boss who you know dislikes and disapproves of you – perhaps you've had this experience. It makes it hard to improve your work performance. For a child in school, who lacks the motivation of getting paid, lacks the life experience to manage the situation in an effective way, and lacks the power to remove themselves from the circumstances, it's even worse. They might react with distracting behaviours, or absconding, or such high levels of anxiety that they have a panic attack.

On the other hand, when a child knows the teacher likes them, they are more likely to respond positively. Our experience is that our children begin to grow in love with a subject if they know the teacher likes them. It's important to be aware of this relationship when planning strategies for that child's time in school.

Of course, teachers are only human! Sometimes, things have been so difficult with a child that dislike – or even legitimate fear of a child – may be understandable. This is a normal human reaction. If a child is seriously violent towards a teacher, there will be trauma for that teacher, and this should not be overlooked. Remember, one of the first principles we learned with our NVR model was that safety is utmost for all. With Ch4, for example, I have often said that I could not cope with what my child puts the teacher through – we have made breakthroughs at home, but his relationship with his teachers is its own thing. Child on parent/carer/teacher violence is rarely talked about, and there is very little help out there. Repairing the relationship, if at all possible, is key to moving forward – and if a relationship cannot be repaired then, as with Ch4, ending the relationship from either side may become the only viable option.

What is the child's relationship with their peers like?

This is another crucial area for children of all ages and neurotypes, but especially as young people move into their teens. Even normal relationship falling-out and making-up can be the biggest thing in a child's world, but the impact can be astronomical when normal fallings-out escalate into bullying. In primary school, it seems that most bullying goes on in the playground, where escape may be more possible. As teens, though, this spills into the classroom, where subtle hostility or mocking can be rife. Behaviours can be missed by teachers, who are focusing on delivering a lesson and managing a room of many young people, but their impact will still be wholly felt by the bullied student.

As children grow into teens and young adults, much of their interaction also happens online. This is a whole new world of comparison and intimidation. If things have gone wrong in a relationship, my autistic children will find it impossible to sit with others comfortably in class.

Anti-bullying and restorative justice

For the past ten years, I have been an ambassador of the Diana Award, a charity largely dedicated to anti-bullying. The work the charity does is incredible in empowering the voices of bullied and vulnerable children. All schools in the United Kingdom have to have an anti-bullying policy, which is usually posted on their website. But of course, we all know that this has not solved bullying in UK schools! It is interesting to look at how a school deals with bullying in actuality and in principle. Most posted policies will tell you they have zero tolerance towards bullying, and list the punishments for anyone found to be bullying. Very few, however, look at the subtleties of bullying or how to eradicate it completely.

In Ch2's secondary school, they believed the best way to deal with allegations of bullying was to interview all the bystanders to find out the truth. While this looks good on paper, it also under-estimates the intelligence of young people to a certain extent. Teenagers are not stupid, and those intent on excluding or alienating a peer can think of ways to not get caught – for example, I know from experience that a group of young people all working out together what they will say when interviewed, in order to support their bullying friend, can have a devastating effect on a bullied child. My less-popular bullied child unravelled at this point – it must have felt like literally the whole world was against them – and still struggles with the impact of the trauma to this day.

Or schools might take an "it takes two" approach to their bullying policies. I remember when two young women had sent a series of videos to my child, telling them to kill themselves and mocking their autism and mental health issues. As you can imagine, this was hugely traumatic for my vulnerable child, and is almost the very dictionary definition of cyber-bullying. While the school did set a fixed exclusion of one week for both perpetrators, we were not told this until later. The first we knew of the school's response to this life-endangering example of bullying was when, after we were invited in for a meeting, the school brought up a social media post that my child had made, suggesting that they had somehow brought this bullying on themselves. The post in question was extremely tame, and not actually related to the incident at all. "It takes two" would surely only apply if Ch2 had been sending similar suicide-baiting, cruel, and mocking videos individually to these young people, with someone else roped in to outnumber them – anything short of this, and treating both sides as being "as bad as each other" is simply not appropriate. We were bewildered. It was victim blaming and shaming at its worst. In attempting to be fair and unbiased, the school failed to protect Ch2 from bullying on multiple occasions.

So what did work?

The young women were excluded from school for a week. On their return, they were told that they were not allowed to speak to my child. This should solve the issue, right? Again, this seriously under-estimates the intelligence of young people, and people's capacity for malice. In the following weeks, these girls would pass my child in the corridor and stamp their feet suddenly as they passed. As you can imagine, this jump-scared my autistic, sensitive to sensory input child. If Ch2 was chatting to someone in the school playground, they would come and speak to the person our child was speaking to, completely ignoring my child. Although they followed the letter of the law as it had been laid down to them, it was basically business as usual.

I wrote to the school and asked them to do a piece of work around restorative justice, where all concerned could be reconciled. I was turned down. I persisted and continued to be turned down, but eventually one teacher said she would give time and space for this to happen. Ch2 wrote what was effectively an NVR announcement. Dealing with each young woman separately, it told them how much my child had valued their friendship in the past, laid out how my child felt about the bullying words, and called on each of them to make amends by coming up with a strategy that would reconcile them.

As the first young woman listened to my child read their piece, it became clear that – much like the instant difference we saw when using NVR tools with Ch4 for the first time – this method had made an impact that nothing else had managed to achieve. There were lots of tears, and the first of Ch2's erstwhile tormentors apologized and volunteered to come to the top of our road and walk into school with Ch2 each morning as a message not only to Ch2 but to all the bystanders that the war was over and peace had been made. In the next encounter, the second young woman had a very similar response: her idea for reconciliation was to buy my child flowers as a gesture of apology.

Unlike anything that had been tried before, this approach totally empowered Ch2. It was a thorough and meaningful solution to the issues between the young people, and ended this particular bullying situation once and for all. I believe – although I cannot prove it – that this approach also meant that these young women will think twice before doing anything like this again. People make mistakes – sometimes bad ones, and sometimes maliciously – but we must allow for growth and evolution, especially with our young people, and facing the impact of their actions in this way is often the key to change for people.

Reasonable adjustments

In school, as in the workplace as adults, there is a certain level of obligation for organizations to make what are called reasonable adjustments in order to allow equal access to opportunities. Reasonable adjustments do not have to be huge; there are so many little changes that can make a big difference to individuals. Here's a list of small things that have helped our children over the years.

- **Laminated cards**. Each card is a 4 cm by 3 cm (approx.) piece of paper, which has been laminated and can be used in a number of ways. In some cases, it may be just one card, blue on one side and yellow on the other. The child or young person pops the card at the front of the desk where they are working. Blue signals to the teacher they are okay and yellow means they need help/need to leave. Ch2 used this card a lot in secondary school if they felt they were about to have a panic attack. Sometimes there are two cards, one red and one green. Ch4 used to carry these in his pockets when he was in Reception year, and show them to the teacher if he felt he needed to. Red meant that he really needed help or was angry, while green meant he was doing okay.

- **Keychain cards**. This is a keychain, with a number of pictures attached that show different emotions. Emojis are sometimes used; these can be very useful if the child is already familiar with emojis. The pictures can then be used by both a TA and a child to help communication. This tool is great for children when they are not so good at finding the right words for emotions. Tony Attwood's (2009) CAT Kit has the most extensive range of facial expressions in cartoon form with pages of Velcro faces. There are 10 emotional states – joy, safety, love, surprise, pride, shame, anger, disgust, fear, and sadness – and each of these sections has 10 further linguistic variations.

- **School passports**. These are a single sheet of paper with a picture of the child, and a list of "things you need to know about me". It will usually be a mixture of statistics and facts such as diagnoses, age, and so on; things that the child is good at and/or likes; and struggles they might have. They can be super useful in a school environment where a child is working with different adults who may not know the child very well.

- **Zones of regulation**. There are various different models of this same idea, but perhaps the most common is by Leah Kuypers; she has published a book on the model (Kuypers, 2011), and has various products available. The basic idea is that there are four zones labelled blue, green, yellow, and red, and each zones has accompanying feelings and emotional states. Children and staff are taught to use the same model and it forms a basis for conversation and understanding.

- **Time out**. When a child is completely dysregulated, trying to make them stay in class can lead to explosive behaviours as they become overwhelmed and near meltdown. Having a "time out" space can be really helpful. Ch4 uses this a lot; to begin with, he would just walk out. In time, he learned to express to the teacher or TA that he needed to leave, and would ask permission to go to the time out space.

- **Learning breaks**. Breaks are essential for everyone, whatever age they are. Adults in the workplace get breaks, either structured or unstructured, so why would children be any different? Regular times when you can let go of thinking about work – whether that's paid employment or school work – are really important. If handled well, breaks are also opportunities for the sensory world to be re-set. For children with SEND, more frequent breaks can be helpful – not necessarily full "playtimes", but just short stops to allow a quick brain rest or sensory regulation. When my younger two children were small and in school, they would do 15 minutes on five minutes off, for example.

- **Food and eating**. These are both hugely important issues for children, especially when there are issues with sensory integration and interoception. Some children with additional needs have problems with food – for example, over-eating, under-eating, and what would be termed "fussy" eating, although this is a very unhelpful phrase. The physical sensations some people experience can be intolerable – I wouldn't describe this as "fussy". Foods touching, foods that don't look perfect, foods of a particular colour or smell, watching others eat … all these things can make eating problematic for our children. Can mealtimes be adjusted? Can a different eating space be found? Does food need to be brought from home? Can a child go home for lunch? Are regular snacks necessary? For example, for a time Ch2 had an early dinner pass – they could take a friend and eat in a quiet and clean environment where they knew their food was not being spoken over or breathed on (a point of anxiety for them).

- **Learning aids**. Also known as assistive technology, there are now whole exhibitions relating to this subject. Finding the right item can transform a person's learning experience. Being able to type rather than write or record stories into a transcribing gadget, for example, can really help. When Ch1 was about seven, they really struggled to write, and the process of writing a story could take hours. The problem was that their creative brain was writing the story at 100 miles an hour, with phenomenal language and narrative complexity, but their snail-like writing pace was holding them back. At that time, speech-to-text devices were not so readily available as they are now, so we would record them telling the story and then they would transcribe it. It took hours, but at least the story was not lost. Today, their handwriting is beautiful, but they still always use the transcriber on their phone to write.

- **Concentration aids**. Also known as fidget toys (although this can sometimes be an unhelpful name), there are so many options out there. It's about finding the right tool – or set of tools – for your child. These can be incredibly helpful with processing the senses, or aiding focus.

- **The blurt box**. This was an absolute winner for Ch3 in mainstream primary school. A blurt box is a container, supplied with sheets of paper and a writing implement. When a child has impulses to shout out – something that can be common in neurodivergent people – they can instead channel that thought onto paper and pop it into the box. This is then looked at later in the day by the child and a TA or teacher, who can then respond and converse. Knowing that the thought would not be ignored or lost really helped my child. In some environments, blurting can be simply handled – in Ch3's current school, it is a normal part of everyday life and not treated as a disruption – but in environments that are less able to handle the interruptions, a blurt box can be an incredibly useful tool.

- **Changing rooms**. Schools are now having to consider how they work out their toilet and changing room arrangements, with the rise in young people identifying as trans or non-binary. The Oasis Academies are taking a very good lead on this. I recommend looking at the report called *Supporting the Inclusion of Transgender Pupils* by the Oasis Trust (2021). It is available on the Oasis Trust website at www.oasisuk.org.

- **Playground buddies**. All too often, you will see autistic children standing alone in the playground. The concept of playtime is one many come to dread. All measures should be sought to include our children with additional needs into friendship groups; isolation is a terrible experience for anyone, especially a child. Autistic children can sometimes be a little rigid about how they want games to go, but this is a great opportunity to get everyone to understand one another, and for teaching acceptance and creating relationships that accommodate different strengths and needs. Appointing certain children to be "buddies" can help. This has to be done sensitively and with consideration to all parties – it should never be forced, as this will only create resentment – but I have seen the technique used very successfully in both primary and secondary school.

- **Do one small thing**. Many children (and adults) who find it hard to order their thoughts (sometimes called executive dysfunction) will become overwhelmed and so opt out from starting tasks at all. This can be a real problem when it comes to study and achievement. When I can see my children are overwhelmed and unable to see where to begin, I ask them to do one small task while I am sitting with them, forgetting about everything else. Most times, my children will then do several small tasks, they will begin to feel a sense of achievement, and the desire to do more will grow.

- **Do one daring thing a day**. This is another strategy I use when my children have isolated themselves in their bedrooms, or are finding it hard to get out of the home, or are struggling to incorporate themselves into everyday life. Success in one tiny challenge can break the cycle of immobility.

- **Medication**. I wanted to put this in the strategy chapter, as I do believe medication often helps our children. There can often be strong feelings around medications for neurological differences or mental illnesses, so let me be clear: I don't want my children's meds to replace working through trauma, and I don't want my children to be anything less than they are meant to be. Medications are not designed to, and not supposed to, change who a person is. Medication cannot, and I believe should not, remove the divergence from a person. However, I have seen unbelievable benefits to different children at different times when taking anti-depressants and anti-psychotic medications. In an ideal world, I would love the world to accept my children just as they are, and make a world where they feel loved and championed; perhaps then, there would be less of a need for anti-depressants. Until then, if you think medication might help a child in your care, then medical advice should be sought.

- **Self-advocacy**. One of the greatest skills we can pass onto our young people is the ability to self-advocate. When we, as parents, carers or professionals, have had to step in and fight for the children in our care, it can be hard to step back and allow them to begin to share their needs and defend their rights. But we won't always be there. Teaching self-advocacy as a fundamental part of life is simply essential for the future wellbeing of every child, especially those with SEND. Unless the world changes a lot, a child with SEND will go through life always having to explain themselves and their needs, and how they work best, so empowering them to speak up and encouraging them to learn how to negotiate are incredibly important.

- **Awareness and advocacy**. Encouraging our schools to make use of the various national and international celebration and awareness-raising days is a great way of educating others in understanding difference, as well as an active way of demonstrating acceptance and inclusion to a child with SEND. This can be the first place a child will speak about themselves, and it can be very empowering for them as well as helping others to understand difference.

There are so many strategies (these are just a few), and more pop up on a regular basis; the main thing to remember is to look for how to problem-solve, and think outside the box.

Learning objective: Wider inclusivity

To begin to think of the implications of diversity and inclusion beyond one child's strategy. To think about how we might better shape the future to be truly inclusive and consider education on a systemic level as well as a local level.

6
The future

There is no doubt that creating an education system that works for all will take both bravery and courage; it takes bravery to face what feels like an insurmountable task, and courage to make something new and fresh. But it is important. When various surveys of UK adults (Kuczera et al., 2016) show that we have a national reading age of between nine and 11 years (National Literacy Trust, 2017), it's clear that we still have a long way to go before we have an education system to be proud of. The implications of an education system that's not fit for purpose are huge. But it's not just reading age in and of itself: general literacy is linked to other forms of language comprehension. Take health literacy, for instance: a person's lack of understanding – whether they struggle because of their reading skills, or for some other reason – may leave them unable to live life fully, or even perhaps to live at all.

So what do we do? Do we adjust the system we currently have and apply some changes? Do we have a massive overhaul? Or do we start from scratch? These are the questions many involved in education are asking right now. As a society, where do we even begin? There is a lot of reimagining going on, and many conversations taking place – but in all our brainstorming sessions and focus groups, we must make sure that, no matter what model we move forward with, we remember the critical point that *education is for all.* Whatever reforms are made, if our education system does not hold this as its highest priority, then it will fail. There should be no losers, and nobody left behind. Inclusion and equity need to be embedded at the developmental stage, right from the very beginning.

Change can feel threatening, but it is something we cannot afford to ignore or shy away from. Investment into our education system is crucial to the future of our society and, of course, our economy. We have an opportunity here to create something of lasting value that will shape our nation, our culture, our sense of identity and our unity. As we gather in governmental departments, in schools, in multi-stakeholder meetings, in Zooms and Teams, and in person, every group of people must be represented. All views must be considered, seriously, without tokenism. So often, different groups have far more that we agree on than we realize, and we must build on this common ground. On a political level, we need to encourage a cross-party commitment to building an education system that works. The success of our education system benefits all.

So, aside from the bravery needed to take this on, what else is required to bring about education that works for all? I suggest we need:

- a recognition that there are no quick fixes; we need long-term thinking;
- joined-up thinking and collaboration;
- flexibility and innovation;
- diversity, equity, inclusion – and the true goal: belonging.

No quick fixes

It takes time to make change happen. It takes failing, reflecting, and re-trying. Our election system works on a five-year incumbency, and this makes it hard for any system requiring long-term transformation to undergo any meaningful change. There is a "God forbid the opposing party gets the glory!" attitude, which helps no one. Unfortunately, due to this, governments are less likely to invest in something that they believe yields little short-term return. However, this creates a crisis culture, where every move is reactionary and looks only to the immediate results. In the last 20 years (at the time of writing), we have had 11 different Secretaries of State for Education, and this creates inconsistency and short-term thinking. Instead of seeing new ideas taken on and reviewed to see whether they work, new ideas come around much too frequently, so systems are changed, and just as the new ideas are beginning to be embedded, the system changes again.

Our government (whoever it is) needs to commit to long-term change with 10- to 15-year plans. When we consider a child is in education for 15 years, it makes sense to have a longer-term plan. The environmental needs of our world have forced this long-term concept upon governments, which are now coming round to the idea of long-term plans. Co-creating vision, innovation, implementation, and reflection is a process, and not one that can be rushed.

The Foundation for Education Development is doing an amazing job, which they describe as "a 10-year plan captured within a 30-year planning horizon" (Foundation for Education Development, 2021).

Joined-up thinking

Our government has the responsibility to:

- educate all;
- provide healthcare for all;
- care for those who need social care.

As I mentioned towards the start of this book, health, social care, and education are inextricably linked – yet these departments mostly still work in silos. We need cross-departmental collaboration, with education, health, and social care working together; and let's not forget the third sector, which mops up so many of our biggest challenges at the point of crisis. Our charity sector needs to be included in the conversation, and charities need to be well funded and valued. Schools should sit in the centre of the activity. Education is the future – it makes little sense to me that although we are beginning to see integrated systems, including health and social care and the voluntary sector working together, education is still missing from the mix.

Flexibility

For far too long, our systems have been inflexible, and this rigidity makes change hard to achieve. We know this from family life, from relationships, from business: the ability to be flexible with ideas adds value to *every area*. If we are to truly be innovative, the will must be there to allow people to do things in their own way, which involves trust and flexible thinking. Being flexible also means that changes can be made swiftly if something doesn't work (although not so swiftly that we don't actually know whether they've worked or not yet), and failures can be learned from and fixed rather than swept under the rug. There are so many areas where flexibility might allow us to be innovative.

Areas for innovation

- **Curriculum**. Wouldn't it be great to build a curriculum that prepares lifelong learners for the real world? A plan that inspires and energizes our young people. A model that appreciates every type of learner, where all are valued, whatever they bring. If we want young people to buy into this concept, they need to feel that they are a part of the concept. Young people should be included at the planning stage.

- **Teacher empowerment**. We need to do more to empower our teachers. If a teacher is struggling to hit targets, the temptation to feel negative about the students who aren't able to hit the targets in their class will be high, often leading to a hostile atmosphere. This is not good for those with SEND. From all I have seen and been told, when things start to go off-piste, the senior leadership team often increases pressure and over-controls the situation, letting the teacher know they are failing. At this same time, parents and carers are feeling the pressure of making sure their child is healthy, happy, and learning, as well as additional pressure that can be placed on them by the school – so we feel as if we are failing too. Creating a highly pressurized environment for teachers will not make them better teachers, any more than it makes students better learners. Expectations are a good thing to have, but when we start to add threats and unrealistic pressure, all we do is create fear – and fear has never been a healthy motivator.

- **Realistic expectations**. Every learner is different, and targets should be individualized. Of course, there will be massive crossover, and we don't necessarily have to start from scratch for every individual child, but learning is about forward motion. If this is happening, then we are advancing. This should be recognized in target-setting – for the sake of teachers and learners.

- **Innovation at local level**. Too often, national decisions made for all schools don't work in different environments. It would benefit our system if there were some flexibility so that more specific innovation could be applied at local level. In addition, many schools have different types of learners with different challenges, and this should be considered.

- **Social engagement**. Schools should truly inspire young people to have a sense of responsibility to one another and to the wider world. It is totally possible to create unity and community with an identity that is both diverse and inclusive, and also brings a sense of belonging.

- **Timetable**. Why can't we rethink the shape of the school day/week/term/year? Four-day weeks, later starts, earlier starts, shorter days, longer days? There are so many suggestions.

- **Technology**. We need to overcome the challenges, but tech should be embedded into the learning experience. This is the way of the adult working world, with many post-pandemic workplaces changed forever. Working from home has created an issue with team-building and cohesion, and of course this needs to be addressed, but we have seen the many benefits of working from home for many. Can we apply these lessons to school, too?

- **Careers**. I use this term in the broadest sense, but I really mean purpose. In an ideal world, these two should be one.

Careers advice and support should be running alongside our learners from when they start school. I don't mean as a way to indoctrinate young children into a capitalist society where they are only valued for their contribution to the economy (that would not be conducive to true learning), but to encourage children to explore the big questions, in age-appropriate ways, from the start of their learning. Who am I? What am I here for? Young people should be given a sense of identity and purpose from the very beginning.

- **Industry and education**. Following on from careers, I would love to see better links between the two. To help young adults grow into their next stage, we need to see businesses sharing what the adult working world looks like, and all the possibilities that are out there. I know when Ch2 asked to do work experience in the music industry, for example, their school offered a placement working in a music shop. This is not the same thing and doesn't give a true representation of the diverse options for adult life that are out there.

- **STEAM not STEM**. Science, technology, engineering, *arts*, and maths – I cannot stress this enough. Creativity is essential to life – if multiple lockdowns, where for large swathes of the population all there was to do was create and consume art, haven't taught us this idea, I don't know what will.

Next to family, school is the biggest influence on our children's lives. School can inspire or traumatize – often with very little in between. When it's right, it's so good – so let's get it right!

Belonging

The concept of belonging is so important. My dream for the future goes way beyond the school gates. It is the valuing of every soul, of every little person who will grow into one of our next generation of adults. It is treasuring their ideas and thoughts and guiding them along the way. It is telling them that they are enough, that they have a place in this world, that they can dream big dreams and dare to step outside of the things that threaten to limit them. It is encouraging them to believe they can be world-changers. It is helping them to overcome any fear they have of difference, to stretch the thinking of the generation that has gone before. It is to live at peace with those who disagree, but also to challenge the status quo, to push back the boundaries, and to create something new and incredible. It is to overcome the lack of confidence and negativity that pervades our society. It is to raise a generation of young people who will open doors for others and raise up others alongside them. It is to teach our children to love outrageously, to be kind to all, and always to give voice to those who have no voice. This is not just the school I dream of – this is the world I dream of.

Recommended discussion topics

Here are some prompt questions to help you discuss the various issues that this book might have raised for you.

Worldview

- How flexible is your worldview?
- How much does your worldview impact your practice?
- How do you think people with different worldviews experience the world?
- How might you find out how people with different worldviews might experience the world? Think, for example, about those who have additional needs, those who are from different cultures, different sexuality/gender, adopted, disabled, and so on.

Leadership

- What type of leader are you?
- How will you use your influence to shape your staff/pupils?
- What do you want your legacy as a leader to be?

Collaboration

- How might you engage parents in a way that leads to great collaboration?

- How might you engage young people in order for them to be included?
- How will you bring other professionals in and help them to collaborate?

Strategies

- What strategy to be used in school really appeals to you? Why do you think it will work?
- How might you apply this strategy in situ?
- If it fails, how might you adapt it?
- How will you embed it across the school?
- If it works, how will you pass it onto others outside your school setting?

Brainstorming the future

- If you could do anything to create a better education system, what would you change?
- Why do you think this would work?

Notes

Introduction

1. Off-rolling is technically different to permanent exclusion, but it has basically the same outcome. It means removing a child from the school roll for the sake of the school – not necessarily for the best interests of the child. This includes coercing or pressuring parents to remove their child from school.

1 The landscape

2. "Assigned female at birth" denotes a person who was assigned a female gender – called "girl" when they were born, based on the possession of female sexual characteristics. Many people retain the gender they were assigned at birth, growing from a girl into a woman, for example; this is described as being "cis" or "cisgender". Some do not identify with, or feel no connection with, the gender they were assigned at birth and choose a different gender expression or gender identity as they grow. This is known broadly as being "transgender", an umbrella term which also includes the "non-binary" gender identity.

3. Demi-girl refers to a gender identity, and denotes someone who partially identifies with a female gender identity but not fully, or who does not really feel aligned with a female gender identity but considers themselves to have feminine characteristics.

4. The figures were worked out in a slightly different way year to year, but we do know that the increase in referrals for the year 2019/2020 was 35 per cent, and the increase in those being

seen was 4 per cent (Lennon, 2021). This is a demonstrably worse gap.

2 Leadership

5. Originally, this slang word came from Black communities, and meant "to be awake to the injustices in systems". It was a positive word, meaning that someone does not blindly accept the status quo, but has a level of awareness about systems and structures, and how they might impact people. The word was then co-opted in a mocking way, meant to embarrass or vilify people who the speaker perceives as performatively left-wing.

6. In this book, "professional" means those professions connected with health and education: teacher, teaching assistant, social worker, SENCo, GP, therapist, Local Authority worker, and so on.

7. Stimming is a shortened term for "self-stimulating behaviours", something that all human beings do to a certain extent in order to regulate sensation and brain activity. However, it is much more pronounced and necessary in many neurodivergent people, such as autistic people or those with AD(H)D. Stimming could look like tapping, flapping a hand, whistling, skin-picking, clicking a pen, playing with a fidget toy or concentration aid, vocal tics, echolalia (repeating sounds), and a huge range of other behaviours.

References

Attwood, T., Moller Nielsen, A. and Callesen, K. (2009). *The CAT-Kit: The New Cognitive Affective Training Program for Improving Communication!* Arlington, TX: Future Horizons. Available at: https://cat-kit.com/en-gb/courses [Accessed 2 March 2022].

Baron-Cohen, S. (2000). Theory of Mind and Autism: A Review. *International Review of Research in Mental Retardation*, 23, pp. 169–184.

Baron-Cohen, S. and Cross, P. (1992). Reading the Eyes: Evidence for the Role of Perception in the Development of a Theory of Mind. *Mind & Language*, 7(1–2), pp. 172–186.

Baron-Cohen, S., Campbell, R., Karmiloff-Smith, A., Grant, J. and Walker, J. (1995). Are Children with Autism Blind to the Mentalistic Significance of the Eyes? *British Journal of Developmental Psychology*, 13(4), pp. 379–398.

Baron-Cohen, S., Ring, H., Moriarty, J., Schmitz, B., Costa, D. and Ell, P. (1994). Recognition of Mental State Terms: Clinical Findings in Children with Autism and a Functional Neuroimaging Study of Normal Adults. *The British Journal of Psychiatry*, 165(5), pp. 640–649.

Barrett, L. F., Quigley, K. S., Bliss-Moreau, E. and Aronson, K. R. (2004). Interoceptive Sensitivity and Self-reports of Emotional Experience. *Journal of Personality and Social Psychology*, 87(5), pp. 684–697.

Blumberg, S. J., Bramlett, M. D., Kogan, M. D., Schieve, L. A., Jones, J. R. and Lu, M. C. (2013). Changes in Prevalence of Parent-Reported Autism Spectrum Disorder in School-Aged U.S. Children: 2007 to 2011–2012. *National Health Statistics*

Report, 20(65), pp. 1–11. Available at: https://pubmed.ncbi. nlm.nih.gov/24988818 [Accessed 2 March 2022].

Burns, R. (1786). To a Mouse. Available at: www.scottishpoetrylibr ary.org.uk/poem/mouse [Accessed 2 March 2022].

Cameron, O. G. (2001). Interoception: The Inside Story – a Model for Psychosomatic Processes. *Psychosomatic Medicine,* 63(5), pp. 697–710.

Craig, A. (2002). How Do You Feel? Interoception – the Sense of the Physiological Condition of the Body. *National Review of Neuroscience*, 3, pp. 655–666.

Department for Education [DfE] (1994). *Code of Practice on the Identification and Assessment of Special Educational Needs.* London: DfE.

Department for Education [DfE] (2016). *A Framework of Care.* London: DfE.

Department of Health and Social Care [DHSC] (2019). *What People Told Us About Our Ideas for Learning Disability and Autism Training for Health and Care Staff. And What the Government Will Do Next.* London: DHSC.

Diament, M. (2009). Autism Moms Have Stress Similar to Combat Soldiers. Available at: www.disabilityscoop.com/2009/11/10/aut ism-moms-stress/6121 [Accessed 21 October 2021].

Dudley SEND Strategic Launch (2021). Email to Carrie Grant.

Duncan, M., Christie, P., Healy, Z. and Fidler, R. (2011). *Understanding Pathological Demand Avoidance Syndrome in Children.* London: Jessica Kingsley.

Einstein, A., (1952). Brief von Albert Einstein an Carl Seelig, 11 March. Available at: https://ethz.ch/content/dam/ethz/ associates/ethlibrary-dam/documents/Standorteundmed ien/Plattformen/EinsteinOnline/Princeton/Korrespondenz- mit-Carl-Seelig/1952-03-11-Brief-Einstein-an-Seelig-Hs_304_ 9.pdf [Accessed 22 October 2021].

Foundation for Education Development (2021). *National Education Consultation Report, 2021*. Available at: https://fed.education/fed-national-consultation-report-building-forward-together [Accessed 21 October 2021].

Grant, C. (2021). Dying to Be Seen: Why Is It So Hard to Get Help from CAMHS? By Carrie Grant MBE. Available at: www.specialneedsjungle.com/dying-seen-hard-help-camhs-carrie-grant-mbe [Accessed 21 October 2021].

Grant, C. (2021). Tweet from @CarrieGrant1 on 9/7/21.

Hodkinson, A. (2015). *Key Issues in Special Educational Needs and Inclusion*. 2nd ed. London: Sage.

Hutchinson, J. and Crenna-Jennings, W. (2019). *Unexplained Pupil Exits from Schools: Further Analysis and Data by Multi-academy Trust and Local Authority*. London: Education Policy Institute.

Kessler, R. C., Berglund, P., Demler, O., Jin, R., Merikangas, K. R. and Walters, E. E. (2005). Lifetime Prevalence and Age-of-Onset Distributions of DSM-IV Disorders in the National Comorbidity Survey Replication. *Archives of General Psychiatry*, 62(6), pp. 593–602.

Kuczera, M., Field, S. and Windisch, H. C. (2016). *Building Skills for All: A Review of England*. Geneva: OECD.

Kuypers, L. M. (2011). *The Zones of Regulation: A Curriculum Designed to Foster Self-regulation and Emotional Control*. Santa Clara, CA: Think Social Publishing.

Lennon, M. (2021). *The State of Children's Mental Health Services 2020/21*. London: The Children's Commissioner for England.

Lotter, V. (1966). Epidemiology of Autistic Conditions in Young Children. *Social Psychiatry*, 1, pp. 124–135.

Mintzberg, H. (1987). Crafting Strategy. *Harvard Business Review*, July. Available at: https://hbr.org/1987/07/crafting-strategy [Accessed 2 March 2022].

Nafizi, A. (2003). *Reading Lolita in Tehran*. New York: Random House.

National Autistic Society (2021). Autistic Women and Girls. Available at: www.autism.org.uk/advice-and-guidance/what-is-autism/autistic-women-and-girls [Accessed 21 October 2021].

National Education Union (2021). The State of Education: Staff Workload, Wellbeing and Retention. Available at: https://neu.org.uk/state-education-staff-workload-wellbeing-and-retention [Accessed 21 October 2021].

National Literacy Trust (2017). What Do Adult Literacy Levels Mean? Available at: https://literacytrust.org.uk/parents-and-famil ies/adult-literacy/what-do-adult-literacy-levels-mean [Accessed 16 February 2022].

Oasis Trust (2021). *Supporting the Inclusion of Transgender Pupils*. London: Oasis Trust.

Omer, H. (2004). *Non-Violent Resistance: A New Approach to Violent and Self-destructive Children*. Cambridge: Cambridge University Press.

Pawl, J. and Dombro, A. (2001). *Learning and Growing Together with Families: Partnering with Parents to Support Young Children's Development*. Washington, DC: Zero to Three – National Center for Infants, Toddlers & Families.

Porter, M. E. (1979). How Competitive Forces Shape Strategy. *Harvard Business Review*, March–April. Available at: https://hbr.org/1979/03/how-competitive-forces-shape-strategy [Accessed 16 February 2022].

Slade, A. and Holmes, J. (2013). *Attachment Theory* (6 vols). London: Sage.

Strand, S. and Lindorff, A. (2021). Ethnic Disproportionality in the Identification of High-Incidence Special Educational Needs: A National Longitudinal Study Ages 5-11. *Exceptional Children*, 87(3), pp. 344–368. Available at: https://doi.org/10.1177/00144 02921990895 [Accessed 10 March 2022].

Syed, M. (2015). *Black Box Thinking: The Surprising Truth About Success.* London: John Murray Press.

Unigwe, S. Buckley, C., Crane, L., Kenny, L., Remington, A. and Pellicano, E. (2017). GPs' Confidence in Caring for Their Patients on the Autism Spectrum: An Online Self-report Study. *British Journal of General Practice*, 67(659), pp. e445–e552.

Vaitl, D. (1996). Interoception. *Biological Psychology,* 42(1–2), pp. 1–27.

Warrier, V., Greenberg, D. M., Weir, E., Buckingham, C., Smith, P., Lai, M.-C., Allison, C. and Baron-Cohen, S. (2020). Elevated Rates of Autism, Other Neurodevelopmental and Psychiatric Diagnoses, and Autistic Traits in Transgender and Gender-Diverse Individuals. *Nature Communications*, 11, Art. 3959, Available at: www.nature.com/articles/s41467-020-17794-1 [Accessed 1 December 2021].

Young Minds (2019). *Young Minds Impact Report 2018–2019.* London: Young Minds.

Recommended further reading

Attwood, T., Moller Nielsen, A. and Callesen, K. (2009). *The CAT-Kit: The New Cognitive Affective Training Program for Improving Communication!* Arlington, TX: Future Horizons. Available at: https://cat-kit.com/en-gb/courses [Accessed 1 December 2021].

Holmes, J. and Slade, A. (2017). *Attachment in Therapeutic Practice.* London: Sage.

Kuypers, L. M. (2011). *The Zones of Regulation: A Curriculum Designed to Foster Self-regulation and Emotional Control.* Santa Clara, CA: Think Social Publishing.

Oasis Trust (2021). *Supporting the Inclusion of Transgender Pupils.* London: Oasis Trust.

Omer, H. (2004). *Non-Violent Resistance: A New Approach to Violent and Self-destructive Children.* Cambridge: Cambridge University Press.

Pawl, J. and Dombro, A. (2001). *Learning and Growing Together with Families: Partnering with Parents to Support Young Children's Development.* Washington, DC: Zero to Three – National Center for Infants, Toddlers & Families.

Peake, A. (2009). Attachment Theory. Oxfordshire County Council. Available at: www2.oxfordshire.gov.uk/cms/sites/default/files/folders/documents/childreneducationandfamilies/educationandlearning/schools/virtualschools/Attachment_Theory.pdf [Accessed 17 February 2022].

Slade, A. and Holmes, J. (2013). *Attachment Theory.* London: Sage.

Syed, M. (2015). *Black Box Thinking: The Surprising Truth About Success (and Why Some People Never Learn from Their Mistakes)*. London: John Murray.

Index